MINDFULNESS-BASED ELDER CARE

LUCIA McBEE, LCSW, MPH, is a geriatric social worker who has worked with elders and their caregivers for 27 years. For the past 13 years she has integrated mindfulness and other complementary therapies into her practice with frail elders in the nursing home and those who are homebound; elders with cognitive and physical challenges; patients at the end of life; and their formal and informal caregivers. Her work has been published in peer-reviewed journals and presented at national and international conferences.

Mindfulness-Based Elder Care

A CAM *model*
for frail elders and their caregivers

Lucia McBee, LCSW, MPH

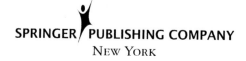

SPRINGER PUBLISHING COMPANY
NEW YORK

Springer Publishing Company, LLC
11 West 42nd Street
New York, NY 10036
www.springerpub.com

Acquisitions Editor: Sheri W. Sussman
Production Editor: Rosanne Lugtu
Cover design: Joanne E. Honigman
Composition: Apex Publishing, LLC

07 08 09 10/ 5 4 3 2 1

Library of Congress Cataloging-in-Publication Data

McBee, Lucia.
    Mindfulness-based elder care : a CAM model for frail elders and their caregivers / Lucia McBee.
        p.; cm.
    Includes bibliographical references and index.
    ISBN 978–0–8261–1511–9 (alk. paper)
    1. Frail elderly—Diseases—Alternative treatment. 2. Frail elderly—Nursing home care. 3. Alternative medicine. 4. Meditation. 5. Caregivers. 6. Mind and body. I. Title.
    [DNLM: 1. Frail Elderly. 2. Health Services for the Aged. 3. Caregivers. 4. Communication. 5. Mind-Body Relations (Metaphysics) 6. Professional-Patient Relations. WT 31 M4778m 2008]

RC953.8.A48M23 2008
362.16—dc22   2007045872

Printed in the United States of America by Berryville Graphics

For my mother
Mary Louise Haskell
Who continues to teach me about aging with creativity,
awareness and courage.

For my father
Weston Bradford Haskell, Jr.
Who taught me about dying with wit, wisdom and grace.

For my children
Cary Paul and Louisa McBee
Who light up my life.

Contents

Foreword

Each one of us is growing older moment-by-moment; how might we live this season of our life more fully? As a society, will we make the commitment to escorting with dignity, high regard, and honesty those among us growing old? To do so, something will have to change. Most probably, as a starting point, our collective denial of old age will have to go—no matter our age or socioeconomic status, what generation we inhabit, or what ideas, opinions, and dogged fantasies we entertain about ourselves, our lives, our health, and our longevity.

Unearthing and slowly dissolving this denial is never easy. It is said that when the historical Buddha, sheltered and extremely protected as a young prince, finally came face to face with sickness, old age, and death, he was struck so hard by his recognition of the human condition's underbelly that any remaining semblance of safeguard from the world's suffering was irrevocably shattered. In its place a radical acceptance—a seeing of things just as they are—dawned, and his long journey toward the release from his and our undue suffering began. Twenty-five-hundred years later, we remain beneficiaries of this stunning recognition and the restorative, healing forces set loose by such clear seeing, unwavering attention, and compassion. While colored in various shades by the diverse palettes of culture, context, and time, the liberating affirmation of the inborn genius and luminosity of human beings is ubiquitous and universal. It is the hallmark of all visionary activity, as true of the Buddha as of Martin Luther King, Jr.; of Jesus as of Gandhi; of Nelson Mandela as of Ahn Sang Su Chi; of you as of me.

Now, with kindred recognition and lucidity, Lucia McBee sets before us the lived reality faced by too many of our elder folk: isolation, alienation, frailty, and the looming shadow of dementia. No matter what our occupation or age, we are all heading in this direction. How shall we approach this reckoning?

Who will provide us with a path, a way of working with ourselves, in the good company of others, when our time arrives? As caregivers—and most of us are in one capacity or another—how shall we work with people already wading deep into this stream? What if as a society we collectively begin asking ourselves questions like these: What abilities do elders actually possess? What stereotypical views do we persist in holding onto about old people? How do these preconceptions shape our willingness to work with them? Is it possible to honor and invigorate the innate resources of people who are living into their ninth or tenth decade? And if to this final question we answer "yes" or "I don't know," we will likely wonder if anyone has cleared a path through this forest before us and if they have left blaze marks on the trees for us to follow.

Lucia McBee has left such marks. You are holding them in your hands, but you will have to enter the forest with her to read the signs and know. There is no other way. This is Lucia's path. As her longtime colleague and friend, I have watched and respectfully admired her unfolding work. Fifteen years into this effort, she is brave, humble, and wise enough to now share some portion of her passionate, clear-eyed journey with us. She began her journey by wondering and asking herself questions; it is palpably clear that her asking is ongoing. It is alive and vital, essential and innovative. Her presence and aliveness make the contents of this book attractive and compelling, startling and unsettling. Gently yet persistently, she asks nothing less of us than our willingness to look unwaveringly at growing old and at our work and relationships with those walking this path ahead of us. Lucia has explored this terrain; in her beautifully crafted account we have the great good fortune to be offered her experience, growing understanding, and yet unanswered questions.

While you now know that Lucia's primary work has been with elders, what is absolutely unique about this book is that she has fused and infused her life and work with the practice of mindfulness and mindfulness meditation and the principles, practices, and attitudinal foundations of mindfulness-based stress reduction. Forged and tempered in the crucible of nursing homes and other elder care facilities, it is evident that Lucia has been *transformed*. Now, she shares with us her gold—the conception, trial-and-error implementation, and initial scientific investigation of a new, educationally oriented treatment approach that she has named mindfulness-based elder care.

This book is her *transmission* to us—a direct line into our hearts and minds, bodies and souls—made possible because she has kept her heart's ear to the rail and reveals to us the sounds of this intimate listening and the actions that have risen out of such heartfelt and thoughtful lingering. She has labored in love, holding close to her heart our Old Ones. Returning the gesture, they have broken open Lucia's heart, thereby releasing her enlivening genius. We are all better for this. I have been shaken and stirred by Lucia's unbending intention, enduring commitment, and pioneering vision. I trust that you will be, too.

Saki F. Santorelli, EdD, MA
Associate Professor of Medicine,
Executive Director, Center for Mindfulness in Medicine,
Health Care, and Society
University of Massachusetts Medical School
Worcester, MA

Preface

After I started writing this book I decided to go into a very large bookstore in mid-Manhattan to view other books on the subject of aging. I asked the salesperson to direct me, and she brought me to the section entitled "Disease." She then pointed out the small selection on Aging—in between Acne and Alzheimer's. These few books were titled *Overcoming Aging* or *Anti-aging*. I was taken aback, having just passed through an immense section devoted to pregnancy, childbirth, and raising children. In time, this same depth and variety of information on aging will be available. I look forward to returning to this bookstore and finding that aging resources are no longer in the Disease section. This book will be a part of this literature. I write it for elders, those who care for elders, those who care about elders, and those who will be elders.

Our culture is in widespread denial of aging. This denial has personal and social consequences as the over-65 population explodes and baby boomers turn 60. We are living longer, but with more chronic disease and disability. Our health care system, excellent with crises, is not designed to care for people with chronic, long-term illness. Nursing homes are the second most regulated industry in this country (nuclear power plants are first), and yet, most consumers find them inadequate at best.

Health care professionals in all settings and contexts have begun to question the way care is provided. Professionals and consumers are integrating Complementary and Alternative Medicine (CAM) with more conventional health care. Nursing home pioneers are advocating drastic changes in traditional models—a "Culture Change." CAM and Culture Change programs and innovations cannot be viewed as supplements; the core foundation needs to be reconsidered. Multiple initiatives are called for; Mindfulness-Based Elder Care is one.

Mindfulness-Based Elder Care (MBEC) conveys the benefits of meditation, gentle yoga, and mindfulness—accessibly—to frail elders and their caregivers. Elders often cope with trauma, loss, disability, pain, and life-threatening illness. Professional and family caregivers also suffer. Focusing on abilities, not disabilities, mindfulness practices provide paths to the inner strengths and resources we all possess.

In 1994, I began holding mindfulness courses and groups for nursing home residents and caregivers in a large, urban, multiethnic, multifaith nursing home. These programs were inspired by and modeled on Mindfulness-Based Stress Reduction (MBSR), developed by Jon Kabat-Zinn in 1979, at the University of Massachusetts Medical Center. Mindfulness is a way of being, focusing attention on our life with naked awareness and compassion. In MBEC, I have adapted Kabat-Zinn's model to elders, their families, and professional caregivers.

Some of my readers may have experience with mindfulness, yoga, and meditation; to others, these practices may be new and, even, foreign. I have written the book for readers with all levels of experience. In it, I share what I have found to be useful in my personal experience with elders and their caregivers. The book also contains frequent opportunities and suggestions for personal experience.

When I started working in a nursing home 16 years ago, I began to wonder if there wasn't more that could be done for residents suffering from physical pain and emotional distress. One of my first clients was Mr. S. He was in the nursing home because of osteoarthritis, which caused him severe pain and an inability to care for himself. When we met, he grimaced if he had to move his hand from the arm of his wheelchair to his lap. He told me how much it hurt. Sometimes, I asked the nurse for more pain medication for him. The nurse would say, "He just had his pain medication; he is not due for more for two hours." I sensed a frustration on her part and that of the doctor when I asked what more could be done for Mr. S's pain. I also felt frustrated and saddened. This discontent, in part, motivated my journey, which I share with you in this book.

Acknowledgments

If books were able to have a godmother, this book's godmother would be Victoria Weill-Hagai. Victoria followed this work from its inception. She consistently encouraged me to write, nurtured my writing voice, edited the material in a way that made it clear and direct, and supported me in ways too numerous to iterate. She saw the diamond in the rough and helped me polish it. Thank you, Victoria.

Sue Young offered skillful feedback, encouragement, and wisdom from the perspective of a mindfulness practitioner and teacher. In the practice of writing this book, Sue has been my instructor, compassionately observing a judging tone, a goal-oriented reference, or an unmindful drift.

This book describes the challenges of aging and of working with elders. I sincerely hope that I have also conveyed the joy of working with elders and their caregivers. Everything I needed to learn, I learned in nursing homes. While the failings of institutional nursing homes are well known to the general public, I have witnessed remarkable kindness, everyday heroism, resilience, and resourcefulness embodied in the people who work and live there. Thank you, my teachers.

I also wish to thank my prereaders and those who have contributed to this book, and to the development of Mindfulness-Based Elder Care. Dr. Jenny Walker provided advice and insight on the sections relating to medical care. Amy Lombardo enhanced the writings on yoga and wellness in the nursing home with her thoughtful additions. Beth Roth developed and generously passed on the anger continuum, forgiveness meditation, midway review, and leadership in bringing mindfulness to underserved populations. Luis Sierra shared his skillful practices working with elders with dementia, and contributed to the handouts. Meg Haskell offered insights on the reality of working in nursing homes and feedback on this book. Diana Kamila provided initial direction on the use of humor, and she always makes me laugh. Elana Rosenbaum, a pioneer in her life and work, contributed inspiration and ideas on applying mindfulness practice creatively. Joyce Hitchcock shared her story on the use of music to connect. Dr. Gary Epstein-Lubow commented on and analyzed results of the Caregiver Mindfulness Group. Joan Griffiths-Vega shared observations and anecdotes on caregiver MBSR groups. Sarah Bober,

Sarah Segal-McCaslin, and Liz Arnone, among other social work students extraordinaire, kindly shared their remembrances of creative interventions they employed. Thanks to all, and also to Sheri W. Sussman and Alana Stein, my insightful editor and her attentive assistant.

My Sangha, if you see and hear yourself in this book—you are! Each one of you has educated and inspired me with your consistent openness to growth and possibility, laughter and joyfulness, intimacy and integrity.

The practices of mindfulness, as developed and taught by Jon Kabat-Zinn, have provided instruction and guidance for my work and my life. The Center for Mindfulness in Medicine, Healthcare and Society, now under the astute custody of Saki Santorelli, continues to be a beacon of light, expanding our vision of how we live and how we heal. And thank you, Saki, for your consistent personal encouragement.

I, and so many others, are indebted to the pioneers who care for elders and the disabled—those who do not accept the status quo, envisioning and advocating new ways of caring: the Pioneer Network, Eden Alternative, Paraprofessional Healthcare Institute, the Zen Hospice, the Spiritual Eldering Institute, and l'Arche.

During my journey I have not been alone or first. Rev. Fanny Erickson, whose leadership in establishing a Wellness Center at the Riverside Church served as a model for the incorporation of body, spirit, and mind in healing practices. Dr. Polly Wheat, who invited me to expand my teaching practice to a younger population and demonstrated the true integration of health care and mindfulness at the Barnard College Health Center. Dr. James S. Gordon, founder of the Center for Mind-Body Medicine, who wisely advised me "to start with the caregivers."

At the Jewish Home and Hospital in Manhattan, I was privileged to work with many fine professionals, and their input into the development of this body of work has been invaluable. My initial social work mentor, Dr. Pat Kolb, also inspired and encouraged me to write. My first co-leader of mindfulness groups was Dr. Eric N. Buchalter. Dr. Melinda S. Lantz supported, initiated, and contributed to CAM interventions and was co-primary investigator on two grants described in this book. Lisa Westreich and Antonios Likourezos co-led and researched results of mindfulness groups, respectively. At the Jewish Home, Audrey Weiner and Deirdre Downes promoted innovation in care for both residents and caregivers. And I am most grateful to Frances Brennan, my supervisor for many years, who said "yes" to my idea of running meditation groups for nursing home residents.

Wise and capable teachers have nurtured my path. I attended retreats at Vipassana Meditation Center under the teaching of S. N. Goenka and his assistants. While they created a solid foundation for my personal meditation practice, the methods described in this book are not intended to replicate these teachings. My yoga practice is informed by the Anusara and Iyengar methods taught by Rudrani Farbman and Rama Nina Patella, and more recently, by Amy Lombardo. I am also grateful to Russill Paul for teaching me the yoga of sound and movement. From afar, I have benefited from the writings and teachings of Ram Dass, Jack Kornfield, Sharon Saltzman, Joseph Goldstein, Bo Lozoff, and Stephen Levine.

I have been fortunate to have Sarah Haskell, Weston Haskell, and Amy Kramer as siblings and co-caregivers who consistently demonstrate a collaborative and loyal family network. Family and friends, whose names are spoken here and unspoken, your support and encouragement has meant more to me than you could know.

May the fruits of my practice benefit all beings.

SECTION I

Foundations

CHAPTER 1

A Box for Father: Health Care and Nursing Homes

A FABLE

A man lives on a small farm with his wife, son, and father. His father was once a productive farmer, but now is frail and cannot work. In addition, he requires some care, disrupting the farmer's wife from her other duties. So, the farmer decides to build a box, put his father in it, and throw it over a cliff. He builds the box and puts it on a wheelbarrow. He asks his father to get in, and wheels him to the edge of the cliff. When they arrive, his father gets out of the box. His son asks, "Why are you getting out of the box, old man?" The father replies, "I will not waste this box on me, I can go over the cliff myself, and you can save the box. Your son will need it for you someday." On hearing this, the farmer changed his heart and brought the old man down the mountain. He took care of him kindly the rest of his life.

How we treat our elders matters. Aging is a part of life. And if you don't like the certainty that your body will wear out—consider the alternative. Unique to current generations is the longevity that medical advances and improved conditions have provided. People are living longer even in developing countries. These changes present us with distinct opportunities and problems. Caring for elders has its own history and can be viewed in the context of health care provision as a whole.

WHAT IS HEALTH CARE?

What does *health care* mean, and how should it be provided? The definition is not static; it changes as we change our philosophy of how we care for or

3

identify those in need. Traditions of healing have been documented as an integral part of all civilizations. Ancient Chinese, Indian, and Grecian cultures viewed both the mind and the body as playing roles in illness and healing. Religion, creativity, and medicine were not considered separate until after the Industrial Revolution. In 18th- and 19th-century Western cultures, illness was treated at home by family, neighbors, local doctors, or midwives. With the discovery of antibiotics in the early 20th century, concepts of illness and treatment shifted. As medical knowledge and technology grew, health care provision moved from home to hospital. Many began to view illness as solely a physical problem, and treatment as unrelated to the mind or the spirit. Medical experts cured acute illnesses. Specialties emerged. Nursing homes offered "nursing" care for chronic or incurable illness, and for frail elders who, generally, were without family support. Healing not endorsed by Western medicine was considered risky or, at best, ineffective.

This model has been the trend in Western health care until recently. Culture and norms are not static; they are always in transition. Usually, we envision the way things are as the way they should be. It is hard to imagine things being different. Fortunately, when we realize that some alteration must happen and that the old way of functioning is limited, the need to change surpasses the challenges inherent in the change process.

SCENARIO

You are visiting your 75-year-old healthy parents. Your father suddenly looks pale, clutches his chest, and falls. You call 911. The medics arrive, begin emergency treatment, and transfer your father to a nearby hospital. An emergency room doctor meets you there. She tells you that your father probably had a heart attack and may have also broken his hip when he fell. She assures you that everything possible will be done. You are very grateful for the hospital and the medical professionals. This is contemporary, conventional medicine at its best. Your father survives the heart attack, but, unfortunately, he does not return to his previous level of functioning. He needs help with his basic needs: bathing, eating, toileting, and rehabilitation. Your mother cannot take care of him, and he is transferred to a long-term care facility. The nursing home looks like a hospital. Your father is brought to a shared room. He is transferred to his new bed and told to wait there until the doctor can check him out. The move increases your father's agitation, and he tries to get out of bed. The staff continue to tell him to stay in bed, and he begins to yell. Your family, already distraught by the placement, sees their worst fears come true. If your father continues to behave this way, you are told, he may have to be given medications to calm him down, or to be restrained temporarily. It is contemporary conventional medicine at its weakest.

Acute care provided by conventional medicine is lifesaving and can provide important relief to patients and their families. Care for patients with ongoing chronic conditions, however, has been inappropriately modeled on acute care and often increases the suffering and distress of patients and their families. Recently, new models of providing relief for chronic conditions have evolved. These models are presented under the category of complementary and alternative medicine (CAM), and (for nursing homes) Culture Change. Both acute and chronic care models are important in meeting today's health care needs. It is helpful to see these models not as exclusive, but as partners to be utilized appropriately.

THINK ABOUT THIS

What have you found helpful, or not, in health care services you have experienced; what have you found helpful, or not, in services as a caregiver? What would you like for yourself? What would you like for your dear ones? How is it different from or the same as your experiences? What would you change?

Health care is more than an abstract theory, it is a service that has or will impact all of us. We all interact with the health care system—in clinics, doctor's offices, hospitals, and nursing homes. We also interact with health care professionals who care for us and those we love.

TRENDS IN AGING AND HEALTH CARE

The population is aging worldwide, and living longer with more chronic illnesses and conditions. Increasing birth rates, lower infant mortality, and declining death rates have led to estimates that the aging population will continue to grow. In 2001, the world's population of people 65 and older was growing by almost 800,000 a month, and those over 80 years old were identified as the fastest-growing segment (Kinsella & Velkoff, 2001). While elders are living longer, they are also more prone to chronic problems, both physical and cognitive. In the United States, 80% of the over-65 population is living with at least one chronic condition and 50% have two (Centers for Disease Control and Prevention, 2003). Internationally, studies document that dementia affects 1 in 20 people over the age of 65 and 1 in 5 over the age of 80. Currently, an estimated 24 million people are diagnosed with dementia; by 2040 the number will have risen to 81 million (Hebert, Scherr, Bienias, Bennett, & Evans, 2003). These statistics suggest significant changes will need to be considered in the way health and health care are viewed and implemented. Kinsella and Velkoff (2001) suggest that "health expectancy" will become as important a measure as life expectancy is today. In Western countries, the baby boomers, a cohort known for its impact on culture in the 1960s, are now turning 60. It is anticipated that this group will expect, perhaps demand, changes in the ways health care is provided. The convergence of these trends has led many health care leaders to consider alternative, complementary healing: a more holistic approach.

Nursing Homes

With improved medical care, elders began living longer in the United States, but many lived past their ability to work and be self-supporting. Initially, elders who could no longer sustain themselves and had no family went to the almshouses. There, they lived with orphans, mentally and physically ill adults, the homeless, and others unable to care for themselves. Religious organizations established facilities to care for the "worthy" elders, those of their own faith (Haber, 2006). Eventually, nursing homes expanded, offering care that followed a model of hospital acute care. This model of nursing home care has been regulated and standardized, in large part due to attempts to minimize cost and avoid abuse. More recently, advocates for change have proposed alternatives to the standardized, medical model of care.

WHAT ARE THE ALTERNATIVES?

Complementary and Alternative Medicine (CAM)

The belief in the connectedness of the mind, body, and spirit is common to Eastern, ancient, and traditional cultures. Western medicine, and the philosophy behind it, is unique in its approach and treatment of these elements as separate and unrelated. Recently, however, this trend has shifted.

All healing systems, practices, and products that are not considered to be part of current conventional medicine fall into the category of Complementary and Alternative Medicine. CAM can be used *with* (complementary) or *in the place of* (alternative) conventional medical treatment. There is an extensive range of treatments under this rubric. A 2005 survey by the Institute of Medicine listed 100 CAM therapies, practices, and systems. Despite initial adverse reactions from some medical professionals and institutions, the inclusion of CAM in Western settings is increasing. Patients, residents, and their families are "voting with their feet" and choosing CAM treatments in addition to acute-care interventions (AGS Panel on Chronic Pain, 1998; Eisenberg et al., 1993; Ness, Cirillo, Weir, Nisly, & Wallace, 2005). In 2002, the National Center for Complementary and Alternative Medicine (NCCAM) found that 62% of U.S.

health care consumers already use some form of CAM, most often vitamins or prayer.

Older adults are even more likely to use CAM. One study found that 88% of those over 65 years old questioned in a large survey used CAM (Ness et al., 2005). Another noted that being age 40–64 was associated with highest rates of CAM use (Tindle, Davis, Phillips, & Eisenberg, 2005). Professionals in hospitals, clinics, and nursing homes recognize this desire and have increasingly added CAM services. They are generally low risk and low cost. In addition, CAM modalities appeal to diverse populations, reflecting international cultural traditions.

CAM models and interventions have fallen into the following categories as defined by the National Institutes of Health's Complementary and Alternative Medicine Program:

- Alternative medical systems
- Mind/body interventions
- Biologically based therapies
- Manipulative and body-based methods
- Energy therapies

Alternative medical systems fundamentally differ from the "diagnose and treat" model of Western medicine. Ancient alternative systems include Indian Ayurvedic medicine, traditional Chinese medicine, and homeopathy. *Mind/body interventions* incorporate meditation, prayer, and cognitive and creative therapies. *Biologically based therapies* use herbs, vitamins, and food. *Manipulative therapies* comprise massage and chiropractic medicine. *Energy therapies* include Reiki, chi gong, and magnetic fields.

ASK YOURSELF

In choosing a health care provider or institution, would you want one that only offered one modality—conventional treatments—or would you want to be offered a range of options that include a spa, massage, tai chi, and aromatherapy? Do you already use vitamins and prayer; do you exercise, meditate, or use other practices that are considered "alternative"?

Culture Change

Within nursing homes, the model of care is also shifting. Traditionally, nursing homes replicated the hospital model of care where medical treatment is primary, administrative structure is hierarchical, care is specialized, and the environment is institutional. Newer models including Culture Change, the Pioneer Network, and the Eden Alternative offer a very different paradigm. For the purpose of this book, these movements will be called *Culture Change*. These models emphasize choice, a more homelike and less medical environment. Care is holistic and integrated. Quality of life as well as quantity is addressed in care planning. Residents and their families, and direct care providers are included. As with other new models of care, however, it is crucial that they not be viewed as an additional program, but as an essentially different way of operating. These inclusive, revolutionary models require deep systemic changes and often meet profound resistance. As with other CAM modalities, however, to many, Culture Change just makes sense.

The values outlined by the Pioneer Network (n.d.) nicely summarize Culture Change:

Pioneer Values

- Know each person.
- Each person can and does make a difference.
- Relationship is the fundamental building block of a transformed culture.
- Respond to spirit, as well as to mind and body.
- Risk-taking is a normal part of life.
- Put person before task.
- All elders are entitled to self-determination wherever they live.
- Community is the antidote to institutionalization.
- Do unto others as you would have them do unto you—yes, the Golden Rule.
- Promote the growth and development of all.
- Shape and use the potential of the environment in all its aspects: physical, organizational, psycho/social/spiritual.
- Practice self-examination, searching for new creativity and opportunities for doing better.
- Recognize that Culture Change and transformation are not destinations but a journey, always a work in progress.

What do these principles mean in practice? They mean that a medical model is not the *only* guide in the care of elders who are nursing home residents. Relationships are essential to quality of life. Understanding what makes the resident most comfortable is key to planning care rather than solely addressing medical concerns. These principles also mean that caring communities are always changing as they reflect the needs of those who live and work there. Risk-taking and flexibility are encouraged. Elders are viewed as whole people, with abilities as well as disabilities. These approaches, ultimately, necessitate a commitment to changing the entire system of care.

ELEMENTS OF CARE PROVISION

The reason that CAM, integrative medicine, and Culture Change cannot be viewed as adjunct programs is apparent when one considers their underlying philosophy and how it differs from the underlying philosophy of conventional Western medicine. Following are some of the ways in which each of these models views health care provision.

Conventional	*CAM*
Cure	Palliative care
Quantity of life	Quality of life
Expert decision making	Patient decision making
Specialized	Holistic
Pathology-based	Strength-based
Institution-centered	Resident-centered

While nonconventional models are not identical, they tend to share common principles. A holistic view is inclusive, and considers healing needs unique to each individual's presenting problem, history, other medical conditions, environment, preferences, and lifestyle. Conventional medicine may have a more narrow focus. All treatment modalities are best used in context. As portrayed in the first scenario, there are times when Western acute care is excellent and appropriate. With chronic conditions, it is increasingly important to consider complementary and, at times, even radical alternatives.

Cure—Palliative Care

Most practitioners no longer perceive their goals as solely curing the bodies of their patients. The majority of health care problems are chronic, possibly life-long, and disabling. Patients at the end of life and their families now have the right to choose to end medical treatment, opting for comfort or palliative care. Hospitals and other health care settings are expanding their understanding of treatment options, viewing end-of-life care as more than "doing nothing." When curing is no longer the goal, healing expertise can focus on symptom management. Conventional health care providers may be frustrated by chronic conditions that must be managed instead of resolved. Success is not so apparent in chronic care, and providers and patients may feel like failures when compared with their acute care colleagues. CAM and Culture Change models offer another interpretation: quality of life is as important as quantity of life.

Quantity of Life—Quality of Life

Acute health care provision has significantly increased the average length of life in developed countries, but at times, with increased disability. More and more, medical professionals view improving quality of life as an equally important goal. But how do we define quality of life? Quantity of life is measurable, while quality of life is individual and changeable. Treatment decisions regarding quality of life are judgment calls. The patient and his or her family must be considered and involved.

THINK ABOUT THIS

What is quality of life for you? What amount of disability and pain would be tolerable for you? What would be intolerable? Many of us believe we would not want to be kept alive by a machine, but would we be willing to be on a machine temporarily if we would get a little better?

These decisions are not easy, and yet they impact daily on the lives of our elders in the nursing home. Many of these elders are in conditions that most people would say are intolerable. Are we measuring quality of life by our own standards? Is it possible there are other standards?

Expert Decision Making—Patient Decision Making

Each patient carries his own doctor inside him. They [patients] come to us not knowing that truth. We [doctors] are at our best when we give the doctor who resides within each patient a chance to go to work.
—Albert Schweitzer, MD

Who is the expert in health care? The conventional medical model often locates decision making with the medical experts. When we do not feel well, we may rely on medical specialists to tell us what is "wrong." Yet, there are times when we know, from familiarity with our own body or from a place of internal wisdom we all possess, what is going on with our body and why. Pain assessment is a good example. Pain is associated with both acute and chronic conditions, but acute pain is temporary; chronic pain can be permanent. Pain relief and maximizing functioning are the foci of chronic care. Chronic illness is more likely to affect elders, who also may have multiple conditions. Previously care receivers were told by medical professionals whether they should be in pain, depending on their conditions, and if so, how much! Newer models of care understand that the resident/patient is the expert in his or her pain and pain relief. End-of-life pain relief even offers patients a pump to dispense their own pain medications at the time and dosage they prefer.

Another aspect of these differing approaches is their view of relationships and professional distance. In the past, health care professionals were encouraged to distance themselves from those for whom they provided care. Think of the professional, often in a white coat or uniform, standing over the bed of the patient who is semidressed and vulnerable. A collaborative approach considers both the practitioner and the patient as people exploring a problem or issue. The patient's family, also, may have information and points of view. All aspects are considered. This relationship is equal and respectful and is an important aspect of the care and healing process. Both CAM, Culture Change, and progressive Western practitioners consider the care receivers and their support system as the experts in their care. There is a team approach to the healing process including professionals, patients, and families.

Specialized—Holistic

Are we a bundle of diagnoses or a whole person? If we have a specific problem, we want to consult a specialist. In Western medicine, the specialist will treat that specific ailment. Holistic medicine views the body, mind, and spirit as interconnected and treats the whole system. Specialized medicine generally treats the presenting problem and may miss the underlying or concurrent pathologies. CAM and Culture Change both focus on the whole person. Relationships, spiritual issues, and lifestyle are all considered part of healing.

Pathology-Based—Strength-Based

Western medicine focuses on illness and pathology. Traditional nursing homes also tend to focus primarily on the medical needs of residents. Persons may be referred to by their medical diagnosis, disability, or illness. Patients may lose sight of their strengths and abilities. Holistic medicine focuses on the whole person, what ails that person, and what his or her remaining strengths are.

In addition, holistic medicine tends to be preventative, whereas conventional medicine is often reactive and crisis-oriented. Conventional nursing homes may restrict resident choices as a safety measure. Culture Change nursing homes consider the ability to make choices an important factor. Choices that endanger the resident or others are not ignored, but residents are more able to live as they wish. Choice trumps caution.

TRUE STORY

Simon was an 80-year-old nursing home resident who had some medical problems and mild confusion. He loved to take walks and would leave the nursing home daily to walk to a nearby store. One day, one of the nursing home employees saw Simon crossing the street when the caution light was flashing. A meeting with Simon's family was called to discuss restricting his walks outside. Simon's family said they would rather that he continue to have his freedom, with the risks, than to be restricted.

Questions: How would you feel if you were Simon's family? Would you want to protect him at all costs? How would you feel if you were Simon?

Meeting Institutional Needs—Meeting Resident Needs

Hospitals and nursing homes are institutions that thrive on consistency and routine. In short-stay hospitals this condition is uncomfortable but necessary to some extent. A long-term care facility, however, is the *home* of the residents. Elders, who have lived alone or with a partner for years, with their own unique lifestyles and routines, are often robbed of these basics. The institution itself may decide much of the life of the resident, such as, when, where, and what to eat, when to bathe and to sleep. Newer models of care place the resident, and those closest to the resident (typically the family or direct care provider), at the center of these decisions. They play a role, with the consultation of the health care professionals, in their daily-life activities and health care.

WHAT WE VALUE

Currently, hospitals and nursing homes value curing illness in an environment of medical hierarchy, efficiency, consistency, uniformity, compliance with medical regimes, and tasks. These models are appropriate for acute, critical, medical care. There are other models of care that make sense for chronic

CONSIDER THIS

Take a moment to consider your daily routine. When do you get up; what do you like to do? You may like to shower, or not, make tea or coffee or breakfast, exercise, or watch the news. What makes you comfortable; what gets you off to a good start, and what doesn't? Does it bother you if you have to wait for your coffee? Do you want to talk to anyone before you eat breakfast and read the paper?

Now, imagine you are in a nursing home that has its own routine with which you—and all your fellow residents—are expected to comply. You are awakened at 5:00 a.m., dressed and toileted, and then, placed in a long, noisy corridor where you have to wait for your 7:00 a.m. breakfast. Maybe, it is cold and drafty. The chair might be uncomfortable. If you complain, you might be told just to be patient. If you get upset, you might be scolded, put in your room, referred to the psychiatrist for medication.

Thinking about your morning routine again: how different would you feel if you could follow a routine in the nursing home that was more similar to your lifelong practices? For some, it may mean staying up late and playing cards, eating a midnight snack, and sleeping in till 11:00 a.m., waking up and having a light breakfast followed by a shower. For others it could mean getting up at 6:00 a.m., cleaning up and folding clothes, eating a hearty breakfast, and going to "work" again. Imagine your life now. When do you get up; what do you like to do first thing in the morning; what is the rest of your day like; what do you like to do before bed? How would it be to be in an institution where it was all changed and out of your control? Would you be angry, depressed, noncompliant, even combative?

conditions. Because they make sense, people will use them. CAM and Culture Change represent two new models in a larger movement aimed at transforming health care. In order to be effective, both modalities must be viewed as a paradigm shift, not as additional programs to supplement an inadequate system. Nowhere is this change more urgent than in the care of our elders.

REFERENCES

AGS Panel on Chronic Pain in Older Adults. (1998). The management of chronic pain in older persons. *Journal of the American Geriatric Society, 46*(5), 635–651.

Centers for Disease Control and Prevention. (2003). Public health and aging: Trends in aging—United States and worldwide. *Morbidity and Mortality Weekly Report, 52*(6), 101–106.

Eisenberg, D. M., Kessler, R., Foster, C., Norlock, F. E., Calkins, D. R., & Delbanco, T. (1993). Unconventional medicine in the United States: Prevalence, costs and patterns of use. *New England Journal of Medicine, 324*(4), 246–256. http://www.un.org/esa/socdev/ageing/ageing/agewpop.htm

Haber, C. (2006). Nursing homes: History. In *Encyclopedia of Aging* (pp. 1005–1008). Macmillan Reference. Retrieved May 13, 2007, from http://www.amazon.com/NURSING HOMES-HISTORY-Macmillan-Reference-Encyclopedia/dp/B000M4QKFI

Hebert, L. E., Scherr, P. A., Bienias, J. L., Bennett, D. A., & Evans, D. A. (2003). Alzheimer's disease in the U.S. population: Prevalence estimates using the 2000 census. *Archives of Neurology, 60*(8), 1119–1122.

Institute of Medicine of the National Academies. (2005). *Complementary and Alternative Medicine in the United States.* Washington, DC: National Academies Press.

Kinsella, K., & Velkoff, V. A. (2001). *An Aging World: 2001.* (U.S. Census Bureau, Series P95/01-1). Washington, DC: U.S. Government Printing Office.

National Institutes of Health's Complementary and Alternative Medicine. (n.d.). http://nccam.nih.gov/health/whatiscam.

National Institutes of Health's Complementary and Alternative Medicine. (2002). http://nccam.nih.gov/news/camsurvey_fs1.htm http://nccam.nih.gov/timetotalk/

Ness, J., Cirillo, D. J., Weir, D. R., Nisly, N. L., & Wallace, R. B. (2005). Use of complementary medicine in older Americans: Results from the retirement study. *The Gerontologist, 45*(4), 516–524.

Pioneer Network. (n.d.). *Pioneer Values.* Retrieved May 14, 2007, from www.pioneernetwork.org

Tindle, H. A., Davis, R. B., Phillips, R. S., & Eisenberg, D. M. (2005). Trends in use of Complementary and Alternative Medicine by U.S. adults: 1997–2002. *Alternative Therapies in Health and Medicine, 11*(1), 42–49.

CHAPTER 2

Learning From the Inside Out: Mind-Body and Mindfulness-Based Interventions

MIND-BODY MEDICINE OVERVIEW

CONSIDER THIS

How do you know when you are stressed? What signals does your body give you? Where do you feel stress in your body? If you are not sure, begin to notice your response to stressful situations in your life. When you experience one, notice what sensations arise. Do you feel tension in your neck or shoulders? A headache? Stomachache? Clenched fists? We all may experience stress differently, but most of us can identify at least one physical symptom of stress.

Our bodies are giving us messages all the time, but often we are not listening. Mind-body practices use this connection to heal. By listening to our body's messages, we are using mind-body skills.

Mind-body interventions utilize the connections between the mind, the body, the emotions, and the spirit for healing. Healing modalities mobilize the mind to heal the body, as in meditation; the body to heal the mind, as in yoga; and the spirit to heal the body and mind, as in prayer. Mind-body interventions can be more conventional, such as cognitive therapy and group therapy, or less conventional such as guided imagery and Reiki. Other modalities include biofeedback, tai chi, behavioral therapy, meditation, prayer, creative therapies, and massage. Individuals are viewed as capable of effecting significant changes in their lives by employing these skills. Mind-body practitioners view their relationships with their patients as a partnership.

Clearly, physical ailments can cause emotional and spiritual distress. We are also beginning to understand the profound connections of mental and emotional distress on our physical body. The National Center for Complementary and Alternative Medicine (NCCAM) Web site lists a number of studies on this subject and concludes that mind-body interventions, when used in conjunction with appropriate medical treatments, have demonstrated effectiveness in strengthening immunity, treating coronary artery disease and arthritis, managing chronic conditions, and improving recovery postsurgery.

Of the Complementary and Alternative Medicine domains, mind-body medicine is the most widely used. In 2002, a U.S. national study confirmed that three mind-body relaxation techniques—imagery, biofeedback, and hypnosis—taken together, were used by more than 30% of the adult population. Prayer was used by more than 50% of the population (Wolsko, Eisenberg, Davis, & Phillips, 2004).

This chapter reviews mindfulness-based practices and programs, which fall under the larger umbrella of mind-body approaches. The skills and foundations of mindfulness practice are outlined here to provide a basis for the following sections of this book where I describe adaptations for frail elders, their formal and informal caregivers, and in institutional settings.

MINDFULNESS

Mindfulness is a core mind-body practice. As with all mind-body practices, understanding the intellectual concepts of it provides only one aspect of knowing mindfulness. Therefore, it is helpful not only to read this book for the ideas presented, but also to participate in the exercises.

Mindfulness is "paying attention in a particular way: on purpose, in the present moment, and non-judgmentally" (Kabat-Zinn, 1994, p. 4).

In mindfulness meditation, the practitioner is focused, but with an open awareness and acceptance, even curiosity, of whatever may arise. This open focus differentiates mindfulness meditation from Transcendental Meditation and other mantra-centered meditation practices. Langer and Rodin (1976) also employed the term *mindfulness* in conjunction with their work, which included a study of nursing home residents. Despite some similarities, there are foundational differences in these two forms of mindfulness, and Langer herself noted that her work was derived from other sources (1989, pp. 77–79). In this book, mindfulness and mindfulness-based interventions will refer to concepts that are grounded in personal experience and practice. The practices include meditation, yoga, and awareness of each moment. These practices often have Eastern roots connected with Buddhism and Hinduism, but are currently taught and practiced independently of these roots.

TRY THIS

Find a quiet space where you will not be interrupted for the next few minutes. Sit or lie comfortably in a position that you can hold without moving. Also, make sure you can breathe comfortably. Make sure your chest and belly are open, and if your clothing is tight around the waist, loosen it. Close your eyes if it is comfortable for you, otherwise, find a spot on the floor, wall, or ceiling to gaze at. Keep this gaze soft and steady, focusing internally. Notice your breath. Is it fast or slow, even or ragged, deep or shallow? Stay with each breath. In and out, notice the pauses in between the in and the out, the exhalation and the inhalation. Do this exercise for 1–3 minutes. Has your mind wandered? At times, our mind may pull us away to events in the past or the future. At times physical sensations may distract us, or emotions arise. When this happens, and you become aware of it, simply take notice and return your attention to your breath.

The essential practice of mindfulness involves being present in each moment. In beginning this practice, we often note how infrequently we are aware in the present moment. Usually, we are briefly aware—and then, we are someplace else, in a flash, pulled away by thoughts, sensations, or feelings. While observing our thoughts, we may also note how frequently judgmental, self-critical opinions arise. Compassion, and letting go of judgment, are equally important aspects of the practice of mindfulness.

TRY THIS

The next time you notice your attention has wandered from the present moment, notice if harsh or self-critical thoughts arise. If they do, gently turn your attention back to the present with kindness and without reprimand or recrimination.

Mindfulness is taught either as a formal or an informal practice. Formal practice of mindfulness sets aside established periods for meditation, walking, and yoga. Informal practice includes everything else! Eating, sleeping, working, or playing can all be done with awareness. Some things can be practiced both formally and informally, such as standing. The yoga version of mindful standing is called the Mountain Pose. It can be done formally in yoga class or informally. (See Mountain Pose, below.) The informal practice of standing can be done while waiting in line, or in any other circumstance where standing is required. Both formal and informal practices foster mindfulness. Our formal practice gives us foundation and insight. Our informal practice gives us ways of integrating mindfulness into our lives. As practice deepens, these divisions tend to disappear.

MINDFULNESS-BASED STRESS REDUCTION AND OTHER MINDFULNESS-BASED PROGRAMS

One mind-body program that has brought a new vision to healing and health is Mindfulness-Based Stress Reduction (MBSR). In 1979, Jon Kabat-Zinn introduced a program that taught mindfulness, meditation, and yoga in a hospital setting. These ancient practices were formatted into a time-limited, experiential, and psychoeducational program with homework assignments. Novel to conventional health care settings, MBSR was originally designed to help patients with chronic, unresolved pain. Over time, the classes were found to help people with an extensive variety of ailments as well as to enable a majority of practitioners to live fuller and more satisfying lives (Kabat-Zinn, 1990; Santorelli, 1999). The Center for Mindfulness at the University of Massachusetts continues to teach individuals and to train teachers in MBSR. To date, more than 17,000 participants have completed the 8-week program at the Center for Mindfulness. In addition, in the United States and worldwide, over 7,000 professionals have been trained as MBSR teachers and approximately 240 medical centers, clinics, and hospitals use this model to serve thousands of clients (Center for Mindfulness, n.d.).

Grossman, Neimann, Schmidt, and Walach (2004) documented over 60 studies researching the effects of Mindfulness-Based Stress Reduction. Baer (2003) conducted a meta-analysis and found mindfulness interventions may be helpful in the treatment of several disorders. Davidson et al. (2003) recently found that following an 8-week MBSR class, participants evidenced improved immune function and changes in brain function.

MINDFULNESS PRACTICES

Fundamentals

This chapter provides a brief background on some practices that may increase mindfulness. Those briefly described below are, for the most part, included in the stress reduction training at the Center for Mindfulness. Kabat-Zinn's book, *Full Catastrophe Living* (1990), and Santorelli's *Heal Thy Self* (1999) describe the MBSR program in excellent detail. Mindfulness classes are never identical, but there are certain core practices. This chapter also reviews mind-body practices associated with Eastern teachings, including yoga. They are often incorporated into mindfulness classes and teaching. Yoga, mindfulness, and meditation have been practiced for 3,000 years. Scholars and practitioners have devoted life-times to these studies, and many excellent books are available that thoroughly explicate the practices I briefly describe. These practices themselves are multi-faceted and are taught in many styles and traditions. This book is not intended to provide an in-depth analysis of them, or their history or various styles. I en-courage my readers to supplement their knowledge by reading selections from Appendix F: Selected Bibliography and Web Sites. The descriptions below serve to introduce novice readers to these practices as a platform for understanding what I have found helpful for elders and their caregivers.

The learning and teaching of practices leading to increased mindfulness are experiential. They are more akin to learning a skill than to grasping a concept. When learning a physical or creative skill such as tennis or painting, one must immerse oneself in the activity. Learning takes place in the mind and the body. Teaching a skill requires the teacher to have practiced it well. Information on stress and its impact is presented didactically and woven into mindfulness-based programs. The overwhelming amount of the teaching, however, is ex-periential. Group discussion and teaching is not conceptual or theoretical; the focus is on direct experience and practical applications. An essential component is listening to the wisdom of one's own body, and practitioners are encouraged to trust this internal wisdom. Readers may have already noted that this book includes many opportunities to engage personally. To best understand mind-fulness, try out some of the hands-on practices offered throughout the book. Learn from the inside out.

A REMINDER

Mindfulness teachings are traditionally viewed as "a finger pointing to the moon." Those who focus on the *finger*—practices and teachings—may miss the *moon*—the underlying wisdom of mindfulness.

Mindfulness Meditation

There are many paths in meditative practice: some use a mantra or sound to focus awareness or prayer, and some a visual image. Mindfulness sitting medi-tation is practiced silently, in a dignified posture, with focused awareness.

Practitioners focus on an awareness of the present moment, at times, a narrow focus on the breath, at times, a broader focus on the entire body, sounds and thoughts. It is not the intention in mindfulness meditation to get rid of or avoid thoughts, emotions, and physical sensations. Meditators are acutely aware of them, but do not cling to or oppose them; rather they allow them to enter awareness. Thoughts about what has already happened, or what might happen, the future or past, often carry us away. Meditation and mindfulness maintain focus on the present, moment-by-moment, without attachment. The practice of meditation is learning to sit with *what is*, and, as much as possible, not to respond or react to our thoughts, feelings, or physical sensations.

Meditative practice is frequently associated with positive life changes. Ironically, letting go of control gives us more control. We learn how many life choices we make reactively. Over time, meditation practice may lead to increasingly conscious choices that tend to be more thoughtful and healthy. *However,* mindfulness meditation is not about goals, it is a practice of letting go of goals, over and over. The story below is one personal example of learning to let go of goals.

True Story

I used to meditate at work with a woman from Korea who grew up meditating in Buddhist temples. One morning as we practiced meditation together, I was feeling very distracted by my thoughts. I also thought that since I had been practicing a number of years by then, I should not be so unfocused. When would I improve, not have the wandering mind? I was certain that my friend, who had practiced meditation all her life, was not so distracted. When we completed the meditation, I asked her if her mind ever wandered. She shrugged and said, "Sure." Her lack of distress was so apparent, it gave me pause. Clearly, I was approaching meditation as a very goal-oriented Westerner. My friend did not appear to be attached to results in her practice of meditation. It occurred to me that there might be a very different way of perceiving this situation, and many other situations in life.

The Breath

Sit quietly.
Breathe in and breathe out.
Observe your breath as it is.
Do not try to change it.
Do not even think about your breath.
Be your breath.

The in breath.

And the out breath.

And the pauses between the in breath and the out breath.

For many of us, the breath is a good place to start as the focus of attention. The mind-body connection can become clear when we attend to our breath. We do not need any special equipment or tools. Our breath is always with us. If we are anxious or fearful, our breath is shallow and rapid. We can use deep breaths to calm ourselves in moments of crisis. In many cultures, breath and spirit are linked, including in the roots of words in our own English language: *inhale, inspiration, respiration, spirit. Prana* (breath or life force) in India and *Chi* in China are words for essential energy and breath, which are linked. *Vipassana* meditation (insight, or seeing by direct perception: a meditation taught by the Buddha) initially focuses on the breath, then the body and the senses. Use of the breath in yoga is *prana yama* (extension of the life force).

Remember the quiet sitting exercise above? As you focused your attention on your breath, did you notice changes? Did the rhythm of your breath reflect your mood? As you sat quietly for a while, did you notice your breath become more regular and quiet? Begin to notice your breath throughout the day and how it may correlate with your mood or surroundings.

If you tried the exercise above, you may have noticed that paying attention to the breath is not as simple as it sounds. Your attention may frequently be pulled by thoughts: *What's for dinner? Where is my life going?* Physical sensations: *My leg hurts; my nose itches.* Emotions: *I am so angry with my friend; I feel so anxious today.* Mindfulness meditation teaches you to bring your attention back to the breath when you notice that your mind has wandered. This practice also asks that you let go of judgments. If you experience thoughts of self-criticism or judgment about your ability to meditate or about anything else, observe the thought and return your focus to the breath. As you practice a new way of paying attention, you are also practicing compassion toward yourself.

Working with the breath can be a very helpful reminder to everyone, even those with many physical impairments, about what they still *can* do, what is still available to them. Some people with breathing problems may find breath work challenging and may want to use different mindfulness exercises. Others with breathing problems may find working with their breath valuable.

Deep Breathing

Deep breathing, or the three-part breath, is a yogic practice that is different from mindfulness meditation on the breath. This practice is simple to learn and a tool for providing relief in stressful situations. Deep breathing can be practiced standing, sitting, or lying down.

TRY THIS

Lie on the floor on your back, or find a comfortable upright, but not rigid, position, with the chest open and the belly soft. You may find it helpful to place a hand on the belly to better note its rising and falling. Take a long, slow breath in through the nose, slowly filling the belly as if it were a balloon. Then, place your hands on the sides of your rib cage and slowly fill it with air, feeling the expansion in the sides as well as the front and back of your ribs. Can you feel their flexibility? Finally, place your fingertips on your collarbone and fill your upper chest with air. Again, you may notice the movement of your body. Now, release the air in reverse order, from the upper chest, the ribs and finally, the belly. Some like to think of this process as slowly filling a glass of water and slowly pouring it out. Remember to go as slowly as is comfortable for you, and to make sure the exhalation is at least as long as the inhalation. Try this exercise for three breaths. Once you feel comfortable with the three-part breath, use it throughout the day and night.

Many people find deep breathing to be a good stress reducer that can be used in almost any situation, often giving us a chance to act less reactively. In the stress reduction classes I taught to nursing home staff, it was reported to be the most helpful and well-utilized exercise. The three-part breath also can be an excellent sleeping aid at night.

Body Scan

The body scan is a meditative practice of focusing the attention on the body. It begins slowly, with intense focus on the toes, and gradually moves this attention up through the body. This practice is used in yoga practice during the Corpse (lying on the floor) Pose. In mindfulness practice, the focus is on accepting rather than changing or "relaxing" the body, although it may be a result. Observing one's body with slow, attentive, nonjudgmental awareness is a good way to begin to learn mindfulness. It may be helpful, initially, to do this exercise guided by a live or recorded voice. Sources for CDs are listed in Appendix F.

Yoga

Yoga is more than physical poses. The underlying philosophy of yoga is similar to mindfulness practice: working with awareness, living with intentionality and presence, and impacting the mind, body, and spirit. Both yoga and mindfulness advocate living each moment of one's life in alignment with certain core principles and values. Many begin yoga classes to reduce stress, and find this path changes their entire lives, leading to changes in eating, behavior, and goals. There also are times when mindfulness and yoga practice are significantly different in their approaches. Mindfulness is awareness and acceptance. The primary instruction in mindfulness is to pay attention, with compassion. Yoga practices may be more directive and instructive. While Appendix A illustrates adapted yoga poses, attending a class with a certified yoga instructor is an important beginning.

Yoga Poses

Yoga poses offer a way to experience mindfulness in our bodies. Yoga is not about turning into a pretzel or doing a headstand. It is about exploring what is physically and mentally available to us and about expanding our horizons. It is about carefully listening to our bodies, what feels right and what does not. Yoga done mindfully is a meditation in movement. This practice of exploring our limits, or "learning edges," offers a wonderful metaphor for coping with any challenge. With time and consistent practice, many find that yoga leads to greater flexibility, strength, and peacefulness in our bodies and our minds.

THINK ABOUT THIS

How do you cope with physical challenges? Do you push through them, ignoring your body's message to go slow or stop? Do you find yourself criticizing your capacities and comparing yourself to others? Do you back off and give up? Are these ways of coping similar to how you cope with other kinds of challenges in your life?

Yoga can be done in bed, in wheelchairs, and with people with significant physical disabilities. In Appendix A, I suggest some adapted poses.

MOUNTAIN POSE

... shoes and stand upright, feet parallel, and hip-width apart. Take a moment to notice how you are standing on your feet. Where is your weight? On the inside or the outside of your feet? On the back or the front? Note any tension in your feet and let it go while remaining strongly planted. Balance your weight evenly on all four corners, planting your feet firmly and squarely on the floor. Feel your weight planted into the earth and, at the same time, your body rising up toward the sky. Allow your legs to be strong, but not stiff. Feel your hips strongly holding your torso. Your arms and hands hang at your side. Let your spine be gently erect but not stiff; there is a natural curve in the spine. Allow the belly to be soft and the shoulders open. Is your head leaning forward? Back? See if you can parallel the top of your head to the ceiling. This is the Mountain Pose. Feel the mountain inside you, around you. Feel your mountainlike strength and power. Notice your breath as you stand. Close your eyes for a few moments and feel what it is like to stand here breathing. You may notice that while standing still, your body is always making subtle adjustments. Like mountains, we are strong, yet flexible.

MINDFUL WALKING

Begin by standing in Mountain Pose for a few moments. It can be helpful to begin with a very slow walk. It may seem exaggerated or strange, and yet learning to pay attention to everyday events is what mindfulness is all about. It may be easier to walk mindfully in a room where you will not be seen so that self-consciousness does not interfere. Walk in a circle, or forward 10–15 paces and make a slow turn around to walk back. Focus on the body walking, the feet on the floor, the breath. If thoughts arise, observe them and let them go, returning your attention to the act of walking. Hands can be at the sides, or clasped in front or behind. Walking meditation is a practice that can be done quietly and slowly as a meditation and also woven into your daily life, at a faster pace, as you conduct your daily business. (Note: for those in wheelchairs, everything can be adapted to a seated pose. Wheelchair users can sit and wheel mindfully.)

Mindful Walking

Mindful walking is also a practice of meditation in movement. Walking mindfully is simply paying attention to the act of walking—walking without going anywhere, just walking. Initially, it is helpful to practice mindful walking in a quiet space, large enough to walk for 10–15 steps without being interrupted.

TRY THIS

Take 2 or 3 raisins, a banana, or any small snack, and eat it slowly, with total focus. Eliminate other distractions—the radio, TV, or conversation. Put away the book or newspaper. Simply eat very slowly. Notice the smell and taste of the food, its weight, texture, and color, how it sounds to eat. Use the direct, bare awareness of your senses in this experience. Avoid naming, categorizing, or remembering previous conceptions about the snack you are eating. Just eat as if you have never experienced it before. What is this experience like for you?

Mindful Eating

Eating can also be an opportunity to practice mindfulness. Eating mindfully is best understood by practicing it, not reading about it. In mindfulness-based classes, raisins are often used for this experience. Raisins are small and usually eaten by the handful or in combination with other foods. Eating raisins, one at a time, very, very slowly, provides a profound awakening to mindfulness.

OTHER INFORMAL PRACTICES

TRY THIS

Pick one time each day that you are performing a routine activity: brushing your teeth, washing dishes, anything, really. While you are doing the activity, keep your full attention in the moment. Notice physical sensations, thoughts, and feelings as they arise. Keep coming back to the present activity, observing.

Informal practice of mindfulness can be cultivated by an increased awareness of the daily events in our lives. How much of our lives do we miss? Mindfulness practice nurtures an awareness of each moment in our precious lives. Clearly, there are moments that are stressful and even painful, but by remaining present, we may find ourselves better able to cope. It is also informative to start noticing how we respond to pleasant and unpleasant events. Notice physical sensations that arise in each of these circumstances. We respond differently to pleasure and to challenges. When we become more attuned and attentive to our bodies, we learn from our own inner wisdom. We begin to note the early sensations of stress in our bodies and to preempt the more dramatic responses to it.

Awareness of Thoughts and Feelings

We can also view our thoughts and feelings mindfully with moment-to-moment awareness. As we develop a meditation and mindfulness practice, we begin to differentiate between the direct experience and the thought or judgment that follows. The U.S. Navy has disproved the story below, but its continued popularity indicates a resonance with many.

> A reported transcript of a U.S. naval ship's encounter off the coast of Canada:
>
> The U.S. captain sees a light in the ocean ahead, and the following radio conversation ensues.
>
> AMERICANS: "Please divert your course 15 degrees to the North to avoid a collision."
>
> CANADIANS: "RECOMMEND YOU DIVERT YOUR COURSE 15 DEGREES TO THE SOUTH TO AVOID A COLLISION."
>
> AMERICANS: "THIS IS THE CAPTAIN OF A U.S. NAVY SHIP. I SAY AGAIN, DIVERT YOUR COURSE."
>
> CANADIANS: "NO, I SAY AGAIN, YOU DIVERT YOUR COURSE."
>
> AMERICANS: "THIS IS THE AIRCRAFT CARRIER USS ABRAHAM LINCOLN, THE SECOND LARGEST SHIP IN THE UNITED STATES' ATLANTIC FLEET. WE ARE ACCOMPANIED BY THREE DESTROYERS, THREE CRUISERS AND NUMEROUS SUPPORT VESSELS. I DEMAND THAT YOU CHANGE YOUR COURSE 15 DEGREES NORTH. THAT'S ONE-FIVE DEGREES NORTH, OR COUNTER MEASURES WILL BE UNDERTAKEN TO ENSURE THE SAFETY OF THIS SHIP."
>
> CANADIANS: "This is a lighthouse. Your call."
>
> (http://www.snopes.com/military/lighthouse.asp)

This story highlights how our observations often generate assumptions and judgments, which may lead to unhelpful decisions. The practices of mindfulness enable us to discern the immediate experience of each moment dispassionately. For most of us, our habitual practice is to identify with our thoughts and feelings, rather than to question or observe them. These thoughts are generally rooted in the past or future, and we can get carried away in them. Through meditation and mindfulness, we learn to witness thoughts and feel-

---

NOTICE

Do you avoid, confront, or engage with your distress?

ings without becoming swept up in them. As we learn to observe our thoughts and feelings mindfully, we may note that they arise and pass away, similar to physical sensations. We may learn to act with choice rather than to react automatically. We may notice unhelpful patterns related to our reaction and interpretation of experiences. Those of us who find it difficult to tolerate stressful feelings may also find it difficult to tolerate physical pain when it arises as while sitting in meditation.

There are many ways to see, and interpret, life's experiences. Our perception of events can lead to increased stress, acceptance, or both. Increased stress has physical implications, impacting our health and our sense of well-being. Stepping back and observing thoughts, feelings, and sensations dispassionately does not mean you care less. Contrarily, being in the present moment is a way to more fully experience it. When we identify with our thoughts and feelings, we respond automatically, perhaps following lifelong patterns that we feel unable to change. Mindfulness practice demonstrates that we have the ability to change and make different choices in how we respond to events.

Guided Imagery

TRY THIS FOR YOURSELF

Imagine that you are in your kitchen. Use all of your senses: touch, taste, smell, vision, and hearing. You see a lemon on your cutting board. Imagine the bright, yellow color, pick it up and feel the sensations in your hand—the cool weight, the smooth or bumpy skin. Perhaps you even smell the telltale fragrance. Now, place the lemon back on the cutting board and cut it in half. Notice the juices and scents that emerge. Take one half of the lemon and bring it to your nose for a deeper smell. Imagine how it would feel to place a slice in your mouth. Can you feel the tart sensation? Is your mouth watering? What else do you notice?

Guided imagery (sometimes used in conjunction with mindfulness practices) is based on the understanding that the mind responds in the same way to a vividly imagined event as to an actual event. Health practitioners, athletes, and others have used this knowledge to improve outcomes. Focusing on an event or scenario employs the mind's capacity to link thought to sensation. Baseball players imagine themselves hitting a home run, or students visualize themselves acing an exam. Guided imagery or visualization explicitly uses the mind-body link. In mindfulness and yoga practice, imagery is not used as a means to escape reality or to achieve a desired goal, but as a resource to deepen awareness.

CONSIDER THIS

Mountain Pose, like many yoga poses, uses imagery to create a deeper understanding of the pose. Next time you are practicing this pose, envision your body as a solid and timeless mountain: your feet the firm base, your arms the sloping sides, your head the soaring pinnacle. This image may bring strength and majesty to the pose.

Many practitioners find tapes of guided imagery helpful, especially in beginning a practice of meditation, mindfulness, or yoga. See Appendix B for more information.

Lovingkindness Meditation

Those who practice meditation regularly often end with a lovingkindness meditation. In this practice, one offers happiness, peace, wellness, and lovingkindness, first to oneself, then to others. Lovingkindness practice is a natural outgrowth of the fullness meditation offers—truly from the Biblical sense that one's "cup runneth over." It also reflects an essential component of mindfulness—that one must start practicing kindness with oneself. Forgiveness and compassion are integral parts of many spiritual practices, and now clinical research is demonstrating the benefits of these practices. Forgiving ourselves and others is not the same as condoning unacceptable behavior; it is a way of releasing an unhelpful pattern. Recent studies link forgiveness with psychological well-being and physical health (Lawler et al. 2003; VanOyen Witvliet, Ludwig, & Vander Laan, 2001). There are many lovingkindness meditations; here is one:

Lovingkindness Meditation

May I be happy
May I be well
May I find peace
May I be filled with lovingkindness
May all beings be happy
May all beings be well
May all beings find peace
May all beings be filled with lovingkindness.

Learning mindfulness and meditation may allow us to become acutely aware of the harsh and critical thoughts that arise. As adults, we often find it hard to be beginners, to acknowledge our learning needs with kindness. As we learn to be more compassionate with ourselves, we also learn to be more compassionate with others. Compassion and kindness are practices that become more habitual with frequent use. Harsh, critical, and judgmental thinking is also reinforced with practice.

THE STORY OF TWO WOLVES

A granddaughter asks her grandmother, "Why do we fear?"

The grandmother replies by telling her grandchild the story of two wolf cubs; one is named *love,* and one is named *fear.* The wolf mother is caring but food is short, and there is only food for one cub.

The child asks, "Which cub will live?"

The grandmother replies, "The one I feed."

In the same way, the practices we nurture and cultivate will grow. Those we starve will die. If we practice love, love will thrive in our lives. If we practice fear, fear will thrive.

PRACTICE

Practice carries multiple meanings in mindfulness, but ultimately, it is simply making the regular effort of sitting and meditating, walking and eating mindfully, watching our breath and maintaining a yoga practice. We are always practicing something, reinforcing it in our lives. Consciously deciding to maintain a mindfulness practice takes commitment, discipline, and self-compassion. Regular practice may lead to results and subtle but powerful changes in your life. Practice becomes your life, not a part of it, possible at every moment.

EMBRACING OUR STRESS

Most of us acknowledge that we experience stress. We are also increasingly aware of the short- and long-term negative impacts of too much stress. Yet, we have little education about how to lead a more balanced life. Contrarily, our culture encourages us to escape stress. Some of the choices we make to reduce our stress, such as addictive behaviors, may offer an immediate escape, but ultimately, they increase our difficulties. In addition, some stress is associated with what we aspire to and value—our family, our job, our life. As we noted in the previous paragraphs, stress is interpreted differently for each of us. What triggers stress in me may not trigger stress in you, and vice versa. Our bodies are excellent stress barometers. While stress may cause some unpleasant physical symptoms, we can use mind-body skills to help heal.

Mindfulness teachings offer a new paradigm for stress management. Rather than escaping, avoiding, or struggling with our stress, mindfulness practice encourages us to engage and embrace it. Life will always involve both joy and pain. When we engage life fully, we may find our lives richer and more joyful. The body-mind practices of mindfulness offer skills that enable us to have those experiences. Over time, many who practice these skills regularly may also find themselves making more helpful choices in their lives.

In this book I describe programs offered to frail elders and their care-givers, inspired by Mindfulness-Based Stress Reduction. The rigorous prac-tices have beenmodified for this population, and I have called my adaptations Mindfulness-Based Elder Care (MBEC). In the beginning, I wondered if a psychoeducational group would work in a population where approximately 80% also are diagnosed with dementia. Would residents be able to follow the instructions? How would we do the yoga stretches? What about residents who were profoundly hard of hearing or those with visual impairment—how would these elders be able to participate in a group like this? I also wondered how elders would respond to meditation and mindfulness. Would the elders find these practices too foreign? How would I be able to find a quiet place to gather for meditation and stress reduction? Ultimately, I decided that this practice was too important to deny to our elders. I also believed that I could find ways to adapt mindfulness groups, keeping the intention intact, and yet, presenting the information and practices in ways that even elders with significant cognitive and physical frailties could benefit. The philosophies of yoga and mindfulness may be more appropriate than ever for our elders. Both philosophies provide a vehicle for deepening our understanding of what is transient in life and what is steadfast.

REFERENCES

Baer, R. A. (2003). Mindfulness training as a clinical intervention: A conceptual and empirical review. *Clinical Psychological Scientific Practice, 10*, 125–143.

Center for Mindfulness. (n.d.). *CFM Vision: A review of programs and activities 1979–2007.* Retrieved September 12, 2007, from http://www.umassmed.edu/cfm/vision/review.aspx

Davidson, R. J., Kabat-Zinn, J., Schumacher, J., Rosenkrantz, M., Muller, D., San-torelli, S., et al. (2003). Alterations in brain and immune function produced by mindfulness meditation. *Psychosomatic Medicine, 65*, 564–570.

Grossman, P., Neimann, L., Schmidt, S., & Walach, H. (2004, July). Mindfulness-based stress reduction and health benefits: A meta-analysis. *Journal of Psychomet-ric Research, 57*(1), 35–43.

Kabat-Zinn, J. (1990). *Full catastrophe living: Using the wisdom of your body and mind to face stress, pain and illness.* New York: Dell.

Kabat-Zinn, J. (1994). *Wherever you go, there you are: Mindfulness meditation in everyday life.* New York: Hyperion.

Langer, E. J. (1989). *Mindfulness.* Cambridge, MA: Da Capo Press.

Langer, E. J., & Rodin, J. (1976). The effects of choice and enhanced personal responsibility for the aged: A field experiment in an institutional setting. *Journal of Social Psychology, 34,* 191–198.

Lawler, K. A., Younger, J. W., Piferi, R. L., Billington, E., Jobe, R., et al. (2003). A change of heart: Cardiovascular correlates of forgiveness in response to interpersonal conflict. *Journal of Behavioral Medicine, 26*(5), 373–393.

Santorelli, S. (1999). *Heal thy self.* New York: Bell Tower.

VanOyen Witvliet, C., Ludwig, T. E., Vander Laan, K. L. (2001). Granting forgiveness or harboring grudges: Implications for emotion, physiology, and health. *Psychological Science, 12*(2), 117–123.

Wolsko, P. M., Eisenberg, D. M., Davis, R. B., & Phillips, R. S. (2004). Use of mind-body therapies: Results of a national survey. *Journal of General Internal Medicine, 19,* 43–50.

CHAPTER 3

Knock, Knock: Complementary and Alternative Medicine

OVERVIEW

Complementary and Alternative Medicine, also known as integrative medicine, covers a large range of treatments and modalities. As identified in Chapter 1, CAM modalities tend to be holistic and to engage the patient in the healing process. These themes link these modalities even though they may employ different approaches. This chapter describes aromatherapy, hand massage, creative therapies, and humor as healing options and CAM interventions that have been successfully used for elders and their caregivers. These therapies can be practiced mindfully to promote awareness in the practitioner and the patient. The following chapters discuss specific applications for an older population and for caregivers.

AROMATHERAPY

Try This

Find something that has a strong aroma. Take some deep inhalations, noting the scent. Is it sweet or sour, mild or intense, spicy or bland? How does this smell make you feel? Does it remind you of any experiences, places, or people? Start noticing how your sense of smell affects your mood and memory. When you experience a smell it may transport you to pleasant, or sometimes unpleasant, memories and associations. When you smell baked goods, flowers, or perfume, does it remind you of other times or people? Does it affect your mood?

Most of us will easily identify a direct connection between smell, memory, and emotion. The smell of food cooking may not only start the physical reaction of salivation, but also it may trigger memories of other meals, who cooked them, where they were, and how we felt at the time. A perfume may remind you of someone and may also evoke your feelings about that person. In 2004, the Nobel Prize for Science was awarded to the scientists who identified the odorant recipients. Prizewinners Dr. Richard Axel and Linda B. Buck established that the sense of smell is immediate, directly connecting to memory and emotion, unlike most of our other senses (Nobel Prize, 2004). The use of scent and aromatherapy can be understood by using our own experiences. Even those who are no longer verbal, such as elders with dementia or persons at the end of life, perceive the impact of the smells around them.

CASE STUDY

> Ms. C was a 76-year-old nursing home resident with advanced dementia, Alzheimer's type. She wandered the floor, often tearful, rarely verbal. Staff had tried to engage Ms. C, a former singer, with music, but she was not responsive. She did respond powerfully to the use of essential oils in a group setting. "She began touching her face as if preparing for a show, applying makeup. She turned and pulled at her dress like she had done when fitted for a costume. She left the group briefly, but soon returned with a bouquet of plastic flowers cradled in her arms—like a gift from a thankful fan" (Bober, McClellan, McBee, & Westreich, 2002, p. 83).

Aromatherapy is the use of distilled, pure, essential oils from plants to promote healing and well-being. It differs from the use of smells to evoke memories in that it is used for specific therapeutic effects. For example, if a favorite babysitter chewed peppermint gum, the scent of peppermint might trigger memories of that person, time, and place. The essential oil of peppermint has certain effects not linked to individual memories. Both responses to scent are possible and may have healing properties. The naturally occurring chemicals of the essential oil are intensified by distillation and have been found to be beneficial in symptomatic treatment. Currently, use of aromatherapy in health care settings is prevalent in England, where there are ongoing studies into its efficacy (Ballard, O'Brien, Reichelt, & Perry, 2002; Burns, Byrne, Ballard, & Holmes, 2002; Holmes et al. 2002; Smallwood, Brown, Coulter, Irvine, & Copland, 2001; Wolfe & Herzberg, 1996). Aromatherapy use has been documented in the ancient civilizations of Egypt, Greece, Rome, China, and India (Lawless, 1995).

Over 90 essential oils exist, with designated, multiple, therapeutic purposes. Essential oils are distilled from different parts of plants, including the flowers, stems, leaves, or bark. Unfortunately, many products that describe themselves as aromatherapy are related solely to the aroma, and not to the properties derived from the purified essential oils. Purified essential oils are generally sold in dark bottles in health food stores or over the Internet. They all have a commonly known name and a Latin name. They are relatively inexpensive since they are highly concentrated, and little is needed for effect. If used safely, documented, negative side effects are rare; however, in my experience, a few people with allergies are very sensitive to smells and may find aromatherapy distressing. For most, the use of aromatherapy makes a direct impact and is often profoundly evocative. Trained aromatherapists exist and can be helpful, but the basics of aromatherapy can be understood—and felt—immediately, by anyone.

The effects of essential oils are holistic, impacting the mind, body, and spirit. Essential oils can be inhaled, using a variety of methods, or absorbed through the skin, using a carrier oil to dilute the intensity. While generally safe, pure essential oils are very concentrated, so users must exercise caution. A certified aromatherapist can be helpful when using essential oils in populations with allergies or with complex medical conditions. Aromatherapy does not replace medical care. Most essential oils should not be applied directly to the skin and should never be ingested. Special caution should be exercised around the eyes, mouth, or any open sores. Most important, initial usage should be monitored and discontinued if any negative effects, whether physical or emotional, are noted. Always keep essential oils in a safe place, away from children and confused elders.

Aromatherapy Applications

Inhalation

There are many easy, inexpensive ways to use aromatherapy. Diffusers are devices that disperse the essential oil into the environment. Fan diffusers use a fan to blow an essential oil, placed on a felt pad, into the atmosphere. Fan diffusers are great for large spaces. Candle diffusers, good for small rooms, use heat to disperse an essential oil, mixed with water, as it evaporates into the air. Candle diffusers are not recommended for use with children or in hospital and nursing home settings. Stone diffusers electrically heat a small ceramic receptacle on which essential oils can be placed and diffused. They are also good for small areas like a bedroom or office. Other means of dispersion include a water spray bottle. The essential oil is sprayed into the air in a quick and easy way. Exact proportions of essential oil to water and other application details are listed in Appendix C. For health care settings, Material Safety Data Sheet information is also available on the internet (see Appendix F). Essential oils can also be applied to paper, cotton balls, or fabric. They may stain, so do not use them on clothing or linens. The infused material can be placed on a table, or attached to a pillow or item of clothing.

Topical Absorption

Essential oils are easily absorbed through the skin into the circulatory system. However, due to their intense concentration, most essential oils should not be applied directly to the skin, unless supervised by an aromatherapist. They may be diluted in a carrier oil for massage application. Grapeseed, almond, or jojoba oils all make good carrier oils and do not override the effect. Essential oils also make a great addition to the bath. Using 3–15 drops in the bath water will provide an effect.

Essential Oils

There are more than 90 essential oils available, and many of them have variations. Information on aromatherapy and essential oils is easily available through books and Web sites listed Appendix F. The following paragraphs describe in detail, five basic essential oils that provide a range of healing options. Many of the purported effects are not well researched, but currently, more studies are documenting these effects (Buckle, 2001). Essential oils can be used alone or in combinations for a synergistic effect. Try them and see what works for you.

Lavender

Lavender is the most general, all-purpose oil for relaxation and balance. It is easy to find and not expensive. In addition, the effects of lavender have been studied and documented in clinical trials. Proven benefits include a reduction in agitation and an increase in sleep (Ballard et al., 2002; Burns et al., 2002; Holmes et al. 2002; Louis & Kowalski, 2002; Smallwood et al., 2001; Wolfe & Herzberg, 1996). It is also one of the few oils that may be used directly on the skin with the purported effect of healing skin problems and wounds. A few drops of lavender in the bath or on the pillow can aid in relaxation and sleep. Some also find lavender to be helpful for headaches, acne, PMS, flu, and asthma.

Peppermint

Peppermint is a versatile and useful essential oil that many find energizing and uplifting. Other reported effects include increased alertness, improved digestion, and relief from vertigo. It can be used for headaches, fatigue, infection, soreness, nausea, and cramps. Users should be especially careful to avoid their mucous membranes when using peppermint oil since it can be irritating. Peppermint oil should not be used topically, in the bath, or in combination with homeopathic remedies. It is a useful oil to keep in the car or on hand for times when you might be drowsy and need to stay awake.

Lemongrass

Lemongrass is one more essential oil with multiple uses. Some find it to promote digestion and to be helpful in reducing stress and depression. Lemongrass can be used topically (with a carrier oil) for joint and muscle soreness. It is said to be helpful with infections, pain, and fevers. Lemongrass tea is frequently used in the Caribbean to fight infection. This essential oil may also benefit circulation, relief from colds, emotional distress, and fatigue, as well as anemia and high blood pressure (Lawless, 1995).

Ylang Ylang

Ylang ylang carries a strong, sweet fragrance and is abundant in the Caribbean and the Philippine Islands. Known for its antidepressant and aphrodisiac properties, ylang ylang is calming, uplifting, and may reduce agitation and distress. Some have found that this essential oil can lower blood pressure, and it is not recommended for those with low blood pressure. Ylang ylang is also said to improve circulation; relieve anxiety, impotence, stomach upset, and exhaustion; and even to fight intestinal infections, malaria, and typhus.

Cinnamon

Cinnamon oil is a strong essential oil that some use to improve mood and increase appetite. Cinnamon's popularity dates back to ancient use by the Chinese and Indian alternative medical systems. Uses include treatment of digestive problems, colds, arthritis, menstrual pain, and stress-related conditions. Exercise special caution with cinnamon. It should never be applied to the skin, even if diluted, as it may cause irritation.

HAND MASSAGE

The use of massage for healing is multifaceted. Touch itself can be healing. The strong or gentle manipulation of the muscles, skin, and bones releases tension and can increase balance and energy. When essential oils are used in conjunction with a massage, the effect is multiplied.

So What Are You Waiting For?

Aromatherapy, like most CAM modalities, is best understood by trying it. Make sure you obtain pure, essential oils (from your local health food store or see Appendix F), and use the above techniques to see how this therapy works for you. As you sample the different essential oils, you will feel yourself more strongly drawn to some oils. Aromatherapy is one way to start listening to your body's intuition.

There are over 80 different types of massage, and massage is frequently used in combination with other health care therapies. It is a physical intervention that impacts the body, mind, and spirit. Aside from its use to relieve pain and soreness, massage is often used to relieve stress and anxiety. Professional, certified massage therapists bring training and expertise to massage therapy. There are simple interventions using touch, however, which can be utilized by the rest of us with good effect.

Elders often experience a reduction in being touched, increasing their sense of loneliness and isolation. Elders and their caregivers can benefit from touch when it is used with some precautions. Gentle, slow massage is an especially beneficial tool for those with fragile skin and complicated medical conditions. For elders who are nonverbal, gentle touch can be a method of communication and support. Using a rhythmic stroke can be a meditative experience for both the receiver and the giver. Lavender, lemongrass, and ylang ylang essential oils, diluted in a carrier oil, can increase the benefits of this intervention. Hand massage is a good place to start since most people feel comfortable with having their hands touched. As long as caution is exercised when there are sores, or other conditions, a gentle, stroking massage does not usually carry any risks and may provide great rewards. Elders should also be closely observed for their reactions. While most enjoy a hand massage, some do not. Some elders enjoy the massage, but not the oils, and others like how the oils make their hands

---

Try This

Use 3 drops of your favorite essential oil in a tablespoon of a carrier oil such as almond oil. Offer a gentle hand massage to a friend or try it on your own hands. Slowly stroke the top and palm of your hand, applying a gentle pressure. Massage each finger, the joints and the thumb. If you have leftover oil, massage the wrists and arms. You may notice how quickly stress is relieved using such a simple technique.

feel. It is also important to keep the massage pressure light, more like stroking than a deep massage. While we may be accustomed to believe that only deep tissue massage has impact, elders and caregivers all report a sense of relaxation following 5–10 minutes of gentle, rhythmic massage on the hands and palms.

In over 90 studies conducted by the Touch Research Institute massage has been shown to be effective in enhancing health and symptom alleviation including promoting sleep, reducing anxiety in persons with dementia, decreasing physical agitation in persons with Alzheimer's (Kennedy & Chapman, 2006; Kim & Buschmann, 1999; Meek, 1993; Rowe & Alfred, 1999). Elders in nursing homes have been shown to benefit from receiving hand massages (Butts, 2001; Snyder, Egan, & Burns, 1995). One study even found benefits for elders who gave massages to infants (Field, Hernandez-Reif, Quintino, Schanberg, & Kuhn, 1998).

CREATIVE THERAPY

Art, music, drama, and movement have traditionally been intertwined with spirituality and healing. Drumming, cave painting, sacred music, and ritual dances are only a few examples of creative healing tools. Religious settings and services integrate creative expression into worship. More recently, creative therapies have developed a separate discipline from their spiritual roots. These modalities have been integrated into conventional health care settings since the 1950s, and the Joint Commission on Accreditation of Healthcare Organizations, the nonprofit organization that sets standards for health care in the United States, now requires the use of, "Activity services for ambulatory and nonambulatory residents at various functional levels as well as [for] those who are unable to attend group activities" (JCAHO, n.d.). This standard establishes activities as an essential component of health care services.

The use of creative therapies aligns with other CAM modalities impacting and empowering the whole person. For this reason, creative therapies have been included in the National Institutes of Health's domain of Complementary and Alternative Medicine under the domain of mind-body medicine. These therapies address quality of life and are useful in healing the emotional distress that accompanies illness. As with aromatherapy and hand massage, certified specialists bring skills, knowledge, and training to therapeutic interventions. The rest of us, however, may find creativity to be an avenue for connection and expression.

Creations, such as movement, art, music, or poetry, convey meaning in symbolic language. The use of creativity is especially helpful for persons in crisis or undergoing significant changes or challenges, when a search for meaning may arise. Art and music can be used with any patient, no matter how ill (Boso, Politi, Barale, & Enzo, 2006; Cohen, 2006; Hannemann, 2006). Elders with dementia may particularly benefit from creative modalities for expression and communication (Bober et al., 2002; Roome, 2005). These therapies also focus on process rather than results. The process of creation usually requires concentration and attention, key components of mindfulness. At the same time, creativity facilitates communication with others.

In a recent project, New York City's Museum of Modern Art collaborated with the Hearthstone Alzheimer's Family Foundation and Artists for Alzheimer's to offer small, interactive tours of the museum, discussion, and creative art projects for those with early to mid-stage Alzheimer's and their caregivers. Museum masterpieces by Henri Matisse, Pablo Picasso, Henri Rousseau, and Andrew Wyeth were used to foster pleasure as well as self-expression in the memory impaired. Dr. John Zeisel, co-founder of Artists for Alzheimer's, describes the responses of participants as "amazing. Their insights are profound and to the point, their behavior shows much less agitation and anxiety, and they are transformed by the experience. The impact lasts for days, if not weeks, and participants even remember the experience long after" (MoMA, 2006).

To date, there has been only one published study of an intervention that combines creativity and MBSR. A study published in 2005 reports the use of a program called Mindfulness-Based Art Therapy (MBAT) as treatment for the emotional impact of cancer in 111 women (Monti et al., 2005). This program combined the 8-week MBSR program with art therapy using drawing, painting, and sculpting. Significant decreases in distress, anxiety, and depression were reported, as well as significant improvements in quality of life and vitality.

Rhythm reflects the harmony of the universe, and puts us in touch with the larger picture and our larger nature. Our bodies are always in movement, in rhythm. Even if we are just following our breath in meditation, our hearts are pulsing and our breath coming in and out. We can participate in music actively, by playing an instrument or singing, or passively, by listening. Music can also be a group activity or a method of communication. Elders, who

---

Barbara Crowe, Past President of the National Association for Music Therapy, writes, "[Music therapy] can make the difference between withdrawal and awareness, between isolation and interaction, between chronic pain and comfort—between demoralization and dignity."

may not be able to communicate verbally due to dementia, have been able to communicate musically. When they cannot remember their names, elders can often remember the words to a favorite song. Musical phrases can be used as conversation and as an adjunct to physical therapy (Tomaino, 1999, 2000, 2002).

The use of creative therapies also includes architects and other designers who create healing environments in nursing homes and hospitals, a central component of Culture Change. The use of a homelike environment, healing gardens, and quiet, or meditation rooms has become part of an environment of care that focuses on quality of life as well as quantity of life.

THINK ABOUT THIS

How do you integrate creativity into your life, and what impact does it have on you? If you are not sure, take some time to engage in a creative activity and notice how this experience is for you. Does the creative process connect you, internally and externally, in special ways? Do you learn from it? How do you feel following a creative activity?

HUMOR

Humor therapy uses humor, and especially laughter, to promote healing and well-being. The history of humor in healing is documented in the Bible and in ancient Greece. Medieval courts included a jester, and the Hopi symbol Kokopelli was a mythical mirthmaker who brought harmony, fertility, and joy through laughter. In 1964, Norman Cousins documented the role of humor as a source for his own healing in *Anatomy of an Illness*.

THINK ABOUT THIS

Children laugh an average of 400 times a day. Adults laugh about 15 times a day.

In 1995, Madan Kataria, in Bombay, India, founded Laughing Clubs International by simply inviting people to laugh in the park each morning before work. Today, there are over 3,000 laughing clubs throughout the world, including the United States (http://www.laughteryoga.org/). Physically, laughter can increase circulation, release endorphins (nature's painkillers), protect the immune system, and tone muscles and inner organs. Laughing also benefits respiration, increasing the lung's capacity and the blood's oxygen supply. Laughter, and even a smile, can impact mood. Humor can also be a means of communication. Laughter is infectious and can create a shared experience between caregivers and care receivers, breaking down barriers.

If you doubt the benefits of laughter, give it a try!

Practice laughing by yourself or with someone else—whichever makes you the most comfortable.

THREE OLD MEN

Three old men were sitting on a park bench one day, talking about this and that. The first man said, "You know, I'm really getting forgetful. This morning I was standing at the door and I couldn't remember if I was just about to go out or if I had just come in."

"Oh, that's nothing," the second man said. "The other day I was sitting on the edge of my bed, wondering if I was going to bed or if I had just gotten up."

The third man smiled pleasantly at the other two. "Well, my memory is just as good as ever, knock on wood."

He rapped on the table with his knuckles, then gave a start and said, "Who's there?"

OTHER CAM MODALITIES

The CAM therapies discussed above only reflect a few of the available options. While not specifically linked with mindfulness, all of the above modalities may be implemented mindfully. This book elaborates the successful applications of the listed therapies, integrated with mindfulness in Mindfulness-Based Elder Care. In working with elders who may be nonverbal, confused, or frail, alternative modalities offer a means of connection and communication.

REFERENCES

Ballard, C. G., O'Brien, J., Reichelt, K., & Perry, E. (2002). Aromatherapy as a safe and effective treatment for the management of agitation in severe dementia: The results of a double blind, placebo controlled trial. *Journal of Clinical Psychiatry, 63,* 553–558.

Bober, S., McClellan, E., McBee, L., & Westreich, L. (2002). The Feelings Art Group: A vehicle for personal expression in skilled nursing home residents with dementia. *Journal of Social Work in Long Term Care, 1*(4), 73–87.

Boso, M., Politi, P., Barale, F., & Enzo, E. (2006). Neurophysiology and neurobiology of the musical experience. *Functional Neurology, 21*(4), 187–191.

Buckle, J. (2001). The role of aromatherapy in nursing care. *Holistic Nursing Care, 36*(1), 57–72.

Burns, A., Byrne, J., Ballard, C., & Holmes, C. (2002). Sensory stimulation in dementia. *British Medical Journal, 325,* 1312–1313.

Butts, J. B. (2001). Outcomes of *Comfort Touch* in institutionalized elderly female residents. *Geriatric Nursing, 22*(4), 180–184.

Cohen, G. D. (2006). Research on creativity and aging: The positive impact of the arts on health and illness. *Generations, 30*(1), 7–15.

Crowe, B. (n.d.). [Music therapy] can make the difference between withdrawal and awareness, between isolation and interaction, between chronic pain and comfort—between demoralization and dignity. Retrieved on September 15, 2007, from http://www.musictherapy.org/quotes.html

Field, T., Hernandez-Reif, M., Quintino, O., Schanberg, S., & Kuhn, C. (1998). Elder retired volunteers benefit from giving massage therapy to infants. *Journal of Applied Gerontology, 17,* 229–239.

Hannemann, B. T. (2006). Creativity with dementia patients: Can creativity and art stimulate dementia patients positively? *Gerontology, 52*(1), 59–65.

Holmes, C., Hopkins, V., Hensford, C., MacLaughlin, V., Wilkinson, D., & Rosenvinge, H. (2002). Lavender oil as a treatment for agitated behavior in severe dementia: A placebo controlled study. *International Journal of Geriatric Psychiatry, 17,* 305–308.

Joint Commission on Accreditation of Healthcare Organizations. (n.d.). *Standards.* Retrieved on September 13, 2007, from http://www.jointcommission.org

Kennedy, E., & Chapman, C. (2006). Massage therapy and older adults. In E. R. Mackenzie & B. Rakel (Eds.), *Complementary and alternative medicine for older adults* (pp. 135–148). New York: Springer.

Kim, E. J., & Buschmann, M. T. (1999). The effect of expressive physical touch on patients with dementia. *International Journal of Nursing Studies, 36*(3), 235–243.

Lawless, J. (1995). *The illustrated encyclopedia of essential oils.* Rockport, MD: Element.

Louis, M., & Kowalski, S. (2002). Use of aromatherapy with hospice patients to decrease pain, anxiety, and depression and to promote an increased sense of well being. *American Journal of Hospice and Palliative Care, 19*(6), 381–386.

Meek, S. S. (1993). Effects of slow stroke back massage on relaxation in hospice clients. *Image—The Journal of Nursing Scholarship, 25*(1), 17–21.

Monti, D. A., Peterson, C., Shakin-Kunkel, E. J., Hauck, W. W., Pequignot, E., Rhodes, L., & Brainard, G. C. (2005). A randomized, controlled trial of mindfulness-based art therapy (MBAT) for women with cancer. *Psycho-Oncology, 15*(5), 363–373.

Museum of Modern Art, Department of Communications. (2006, January 24). *The Museum of Modern Art offers interactive program for people with Alzheimer's: "Meet me at MoMA" New York.* Retrieved August 18, 2007, from http://moma.org/about_moma/press/2006/alzheimersMainSite.pdf

Nobel Prize. (2004, October 4). *The Nobel Assembly at Karolinska Institutet has today decided to award the Nobel Prize in Physiology or Medicine for 2004 jointly to Richard Axel and Linda B. Buck.* Retrieved September 13, 2007, from http://nobelprize.org/nobel_prizes/medicine/laureates/2004/press.html

Roome, D. R. (2005, March 11). Painting memories: Art is therapy for Alzheimer's patients. *Mountain View Voice.* Retrieved August 9, 2007, from http://www.mv-voice.com/morgue/2005/2005_03_11.alzheime.shtml

Rowe, M., & Alfred, D. (1999). The effectiveness of slow stroke massage in diffusing agitated behaviors in individuals with Alzheimer's disease. *Journal of Gerontological Nursing, 25*(60), 22–34.

Smallwood, J., Brown, R., Coulter, F., Irvine, E., & Copland, C. (2001). Aromatherapy and behavior disturbances in dementia: A randomized controlled trial. *International Journal of Geriatric Psychiatry, 16,* 1010–1013.

Snyder, M., Egan, E. C., & Burns, K. R. (1995). Efficacy of hand massage in decreasing agitation behaviors associated with care activities in persons with dementia. *Geriatric Nursing, 16*(2), 60–63.

Tomaino, C. M. (1999). Active music therapy approaches for neurologically impaired patients. In C. D. Maranto (Ed.), *Music therapy and medicine: Theoretical and clinical applications* (pp. 115–122). Silver Spring, MD: American Music Therapy Association.

Tomaino, C. M. (2000). Working with images and recollection with elderly patients. In D. Aldridge (Ed.), *Music therapy in dementia care.* London: Jessica Kingsley. 195–211.

Tomaino, C. M. (2002). How music can reach the silenced brain. *Cerebrum, 4*(1), 22–33.

Wolfe, N., & Herzberg, J. (1996). Can aromatherapy oils promote sleep in severely demented patients? *International Journal of Geriatric Psychiatry, 11,* 926–927.

SECTION II

Practical Applications of Mindfulness-Based Elder Care for Frail Elders

Meadowbrook Nursing Home

—By Alice N. Persons

On our last visit, when Lucy was fifteen
And getting creaky herself,
One of the nurses said to me,
"Why don't you take the cat to Mrs. Harris' room
—poor thing lost her leg to diabetes last fall—
she's ninety, and blind, and no one comes to see her."
The door was open. I asked the tiny woman in the bed
if she would like me to bring Lucy in, and she turned her head
toward us. "Oh, yes, I want to touch her."
"I had a cat called Lily—she was so pretty, all white.
She was with me for twenty years, after my husband died too.
She slept with me every night—I loved her very much.
It's hard, in here, since I can't get around."
Lucy was settling in on the bed.
"You won't believe it, but I used to love to dance.
I was a fool for it! I even won contests.
I wish I had danced more.
It's funny, what you miss when everything . . . is gone."
This last was a murmur. She'd fallen asleep.
I lifted the cat
from the bed, tiptoed out, and drove home.
I tried to do some desk work
but couldn't focus.
I went downstairs, pulled the shades,
put on Tina Turner
and cranked it up loud
and I danced.
I danced.

CHAPTER 4

The Sound of One Hand Clapping: Mindfulness-Based Elder Care

THE SOUND OF ONE HAND CLAPPING

As abilities change, our lives also change in large and small ways. During one group for residents, a woman said that since she could only use one side of her body, it made her very sad that she could not clap her hands in appreciation for a recent performance in the nursing home. Other group members began to share ways they had learned to clap with one hand. One resident clapped her hand against her pocketbook. Others clapped their hands on the sides of their chairs or their laps. What a wonderful moment. I learned that small things, like being able to clap our hands, or not, can make big differences. I was awed by the resilience, resourcefulness, and ingenuity of the elders. I also witnessed elders aiding and supporting each other.

TEACHING MINDFULNESS TO ELDERS

Mindfulness is described as a way of paying attention, and the assumption is often that it is a skill of the mind. I believe it is a practice of the mind, body, and heart. Mindfulness-Based Stress Reduction (MBSR) has been taught to those who could understand and follow instructions, had a good attention span, could make a commitment to attend classes and do homework, and could participate in some form of exercise. In this section, I share Mindfulness-Based Elder Care, mindfulness practices taught to frail elders with a variety of conditions and in a variety of settings. While this population does not meet the criteria for MBSR students, elders can benefit from adaptations to the model. Despite different abilities, elders continue to have much to teach us.

THINK ABOUT THIS

You live in a world where everything is set up for people who are blind. There are no lights; books and signs are all in Braille. Who would be disabled, you or the person without vision?

In 1993, when I began working in the nursing home, I noted that the elders there had significant chronic pain and emotional distress. At that time, pain was not regularly assessed, and pain treatment was pharmacological. Emotional problems, such as depression and anxiety, were also treated pharmacologically and by traditional group and individual therapy. In 1994, I began offering groups and individual work that adapted the principles of Mindfulness-Based Stress Reduction to frail elders and their caregivers, adjusting and modifying the skills, and maintaining the integrity and core of the practice.

WHAT ARE THE ISSUES?

Populations are living longer, but with more disability, chronic conditions, and pain. Landi et al. (2001) analyzed data from 1341 community dwelling elders over 65 and found that from 39–41% reported daily pain. Institutionalized elders are even more frequently at risk for pain. Ferrell, Ferrell, and Osterweil reported in 1990 that in one nursing home, 71% of the residents were found to experience at least one pain complaint, and 34% reported constant pain. Fox, Raina, and Jadad (1999) reviewed studies from 14 nursing homes and found prevalence of pain in residents from 27% to 83%. Elders in nursing homes are also more likely to lose family and friends, life roles, and possessions, leading to emotional problems (Cohen-Mansfield & Marx, 1993; Parmelee, Katz, & Lawton, 1991). Recent U.S. statistics have found major depression in 1–5% of community dwelling elders, but over 13.5% in elders who require home health care, and 11.5% in elder hospital patients (Hybels & Blazer, 2003).

Losses increase exponentially as we age. Loss of health may lead to loss of independence. Loss of family and friends may increase isolation. Loss of role and productivity may lead to lowered self-esteem. Loss of home and possessions may lead to loss of identity and even increased confusion. Loss of physical senses, such as vision, may lead to decrease in previously enjoyed pleasures, such as reading or painting. Each loss may also cause an elder to relive previous losses. Elders often live in chronic awareness of impermanence and loss, seeking meaning and stability. "Growth at this stage occurs by integration rather than expansion, and is concerned with the constant imperative to seek out the meaning of life and affirm its value, even in the face of life's impending termination" (Orr, 1986, p. 327).

For older adults and those who care for them, quality of life has become as important as quantity of life. Medical and pharmacological interventions can be helpful, but may also carry unwanted side effects. For these and other reasons, many are turning to Complementary and Alternative Medicine (CAM) modalities, most frequently, to mind-body interventions. Studies report increasing use of mind-body medicine, often meditation, imagery, and yoga, among older adults in the United States (Grzywacz, Suerken, Quandt, Bell, Lang, & Arcury, 2006; Ness, Cirillo, Weir, Nisly, & Wallace, 2005; Tilden, Drach, & Tolle, 2004; Wolsko, Eisenberg, Davis, & Phillips, 2004). Moreover, mindfulness practice has a demonstrated acceptability with elders and their caregivers (Lynch, Morse, Mendelson, & Robins, 2003; McBee, 2004; McBee, Westreich, & Likourezos, 2004; Smith, 2004, 2006). Other studies have documented positive effects of yoga and meditation on elders with dementia (Lantz, Buchalter, & McBee, 1997; Shalek & Doyle, 1997).

CLINICAL WORK WITH OLDER ADULTS

General Comments

Both group work and individual counseling can provide support and insight for elders as they cope with challenges. This section iterates group and individual models of mindfulness practice to older adults in and outside of the nursing home. Elders age uniquely, some maintaining vitality until they are of the oldest-old (85 years or older) and others, afflicted with physical and cognitive ailments, as the young-old (65–75 years old). Clearly, elders are individuals, and generalizations can be misleading. Despite this, a body of research and anecdotal evidence has identified best clinical practices for individual and group work with this population. The following highlights garnered knowledge about working with elders in groups:

- The current cohort of elders is less emotionally expressive. Sharing emotions is not the norm for them. The next generation of elders will have an increased comfort level with sharing feelings and with the language of emotions.
- Residents in institutional settings possess a wide range of differences and abilities. An ambulatory elder with confusion may room with an elder who is cognitively intact but profoundly deaf and nonambulatory.

- Elders may have difficulty participating in groups equally due to physical, cognitive, and communication frailties.
- Fear of loss may lead to reluctance to form new relationships. On the other hand, group work can address the isolation many elders feel even in congregate settings.
- Elders, especially frail elders, are more responsive to directives or clear questions rather than open-ended questions.
- Passive involvement is enough for some frail elders.
- Although elders may be less likely to interact with other group members or to form strong bonds, they may feel connected nonetheless due to shared experiences. The group format can provide a safe and non-threatening environment to connect with others. While the elders may appear less connected, bonds formed in the group may be profoundly meaningful to the members.
- Lack of consistent attendance in groups may be problematic. Elders may not attend due to illness, frailty, transportation problems, or forgetfulness. Group cohesion may be more difficult to maintain with irregular attendance and elders' reluctance to engage interpersonally.
- Elders tend to be more respectful of authority, and in groups may defer to the group leader rather than engage in interpersonal discussion. This situation may change as baby boomers become elders!
- Elders experience a decrease in stamina and a slowing of reaction time. Long groups may be too tiring and defeat the good effects.
- Psychoeducational groups may require great reinforcement of skills and techniques. (Hooyman & Kiyak, 1988; Toseland, 1995)

Role of the Geriatric Clinician

Geriatric clinicians and caregivers are obliged to be aware of ageism and stereotyping of elders. There are, however, guiding principles that may be helpful in working with elders in groups or individually. Group leaders may need to:

- Be vigilant in ensuring participation from all members.
- Be careful of assumptions—elders may not acknowledge that they have not heard or understood.
- For the vision and hearing impaired, get up close, demonstrate, use hands-on.
- Let go of expectations.
- Offer frequent encouragement.
- Go slow.

- Be playful, the lightness of the group leader encourages others. Don't take yourself seriously. Our moods are contagious.
- Use less explaining and more modeling. Use hands-on touch in demonstrating some of the exercises. (Fisher, 1995)

Clinicians can best aid frail elder clients by:

- Evidencing an ability to tolerate their own discomfort with the charged topics of illness, loss, and death; and to be willing to discuss them comfortably with elders, as appropriate.
- Letting go of the need to fix or cure.
- Reminding elders of their strengths and abilities.
- Holding realistic expectations and being aware of small shifts.

And in psychoeducational group settings by:

- Making 1:1 contact with each group member.
- Ensuring inclusion of all group members. This may mean repeating what a soft-spoken group member has shared for the hard-of-hearing group member. This may also mean modeling compassion for all when group members express anger with demented peers.
- Checking in with all group members, verbally and nonverbally, to ensure understanding of the group process and practices.
- Being more directive and concrete.

OVERVIEW OF MBEC GROUPS

A primary premise of mindfulness is that we all suffer from pain and stress and that we all hold tremendous potential for healing within ourselves. We learn that there is more right with us than wrong. For frail elders, this message can be an important source of relief. Most elders, especially, institutionalized elders, feel powerless and disengaged from their treatment. By practicing mindfulness, elders can become an essential part of their own healing.

Recent research has disputed outdated theories that cognition cannot be repaired or retrained in elders. The brain has been shown to not only regrow damaged areas, but also to usurp new areas as needed for growth (Begley, 2007). Mindfulness groups offer a unique model targeting issues that frequently impact elders. Elders experience higher levels of depression, especially elders in nursing homes. Mindfulness practice has been demonstrated to prevent relapse in those with depression (Segal, Williams, & Teasdale,

2002). Elders fall more frequently and movement can improve their strength and gait, as well as reduce pain (Hartshorn, Delage, Field, & Olds, 2001). Research has shown that exercise, even moderate exercise, can impact important conditions for elders: exercise has been demonstrated to prevent or delay osteoporosis (Wolff, van Croonenborg, Kemper, Kostense, & Twisk, 1999), and was shown to delay onset of dementia and Alzheimer's disease, and improve thinking skills in those already diagnosed (Larson et al., 2004). Spiritual crises may be more common in elders due to loss and profound life issues. Meditation can offer solace and a pathway to spiritual roots. Mindfulness-Based Elder Care focuses on strengths and abilities to empower the frailest elders. The inclusion of expressive therapies may also allow elders to connect with deep feelings and emotions and provide a venue for self-expression. Creative arts in a supportive, nonjudgmental environment can foster transcendence and absorption in the present moment.

I offer Mindfulness-Based Elder Care in the nursing home in groups for residents, for residents with dementia, and individually for elders who cannot attend groups. In addition, I have offered programs by telephone for homebound elders, and used CDs to access others who are homebound. The following chapters detail each of these programs. The final chapter discusses the use of creativity as a medium for expression and connection, and the synchronicity of mindfulness and the creative process.

CONSIDER THIS

In the nursing home, an important social work intervention is to work with residents and families during the process of admission. I was aware of how stressful admission to the nursing home could be. Some residents were angry, saying that this was the worst thing that had ever happened to them. Others were more accepting, not necessarily overjoyed that their disability required nursing home care, but not overwhelmingly upset. Some new residents were even grateful for the care and the safe environment. Over time, I noted that the residents who thought the nursing home was the worst place in the world often found it so, while those who were more accepting found the nursing home acceptable and even enjoyable at times. While some residents were able to modify their opinions and adjust, usually their expectations matched their perceived outcome. The nursing home was the same building, the same staff, the same treatments and activities—the only difference was in the attitudes and perceptions of the new residents.

REFERENCES

Begley, S. (2007). *Train your mind, change your brain: How a new science reveals our extraordinary potential to transform ourselves.* New York: Ballantine.

Cohen-Mansfield, J., & Marx, M. (1993). Pain and depression in the nursing home: Corroborating results. *Journal of Gerontology, 53B*(1), 96–97.

Ferrell, B. A., Ferrell, B. R., & Osterweil, D. (1990). Pain in the nursing home. *Journal of the American Geriatric Society, 38,* 409–414.

Fisher, P. P. (1995). *More than movement for fit to frail older adults: Creative activities for the body, mind, and spirit.* Baltimore: Health Professionals.

Fox, P. L., Raina, P., & Jadad, A. R. (1999). Prevalence and treatment of pain in older adults in nursing homes and other long-term care institutions: A systemic review. *Canadian Medical Association Journal, 160*(3), 329–333.

Grzywacz, J. G., Suerken, C. K., Quandt, S. A., Bell, R. A., Lang, W., & Arcury, T. A. (2006). Older adults' use of complementary and alternative medicine for mental health: Findings from the 2002 National Health Interview Study. *The Journal of Alternative and Complementary Medicine, 12*(5), 467–473.

Hartshorn, K., Delage, J., Field, T., & Olds, L. (2001). Senior citizens benefit from movement therapy. *Journal of Bodywork and Movement Therapies, 5,* 1–5.

Hooyman, N. R., & Kiyak, H. A. (1988). *Social gerontology: A multidisciplinary perspective.* Boston: Allen and Bacon.

Hybels, C. F., & Blazer, D. G. (2003). Epidemiology of late-life mental disorders. *Clinics in Geriatric Medicine, 19,* 663–696.

Landi, F., Onder, G., Cesari, M., Gambassi, G., Steel, K., Russo, A., Lattanzio, F., & Bernabei, R. (2001). Pain management in frail, community-living elderly patients. *Archives of Internal Medicine, 181*(22), 2721–2724.

Lantz, M. S., Buchalter, E. N., & McBee, L. (1997). The Wellness Group: A novel intervention for coping with disruptive behavior in elderly nursing home residents. *The Gerontologist, 37*(4), 551–555.

Larson, E. B., Shadlen, M. F., Wang, L., McCormick, W. C., Bowen, J. D., Teri, L., & Kukull, W. A. (2004). Survival after initial diagnosis of Alzheimer disease. *Annals of Internal Medicine, 140*(7), 501–509.

Lynch, T. R., Morse, J., Mendelson, T., & Robin, C. (2003). Dialectical behavior therapy for depressed older adults: A randomized pilot study. *American Journal of Geriatric Psychiatry, 11,* 33–45.

McBee, L. (2004). Mindfulness practice with the frail elderly and their caregivers: Changing the practitioner-patient relationship. *Topics in Geriatric Rehabilitation, 19*(4), 257–264.

McBee, L., Westreich, L., & Likourezos, A. (2004). A psychoeducational relaxation group for pain and stress management in the nursing home. *Journal of Social Work in Long-Term Care, 3*(1), 15–28.

Ness, J., Cirillo, D. J., Weir, D. R., Nisly, N. L., & Wallace, R. B. (2005). Use of complementary medicine in older Americans: Results from the retirement study. *The Gerontologist, 45*(4), 516–524.

Orr, A. (1986). Dealing with the death of a group member: Visually impaired elderly in the community. In A. Gitterman & L. Shulman (Eds.), *Mutual aid groups and the life cycle* (pp. 315–332). Itasca, IL: F. E. Peacock.

Parmelee, P.A., Katz, I. R., & Lawton, M. P. (1991). The relation of pain to depression among institutionalized aged. *Journal of Gerontology, 46,* 15–21.

Segal, Z. V., Williams, J. M. G., & Teasdale, J. D. (2002). *Mindfulness-based cognitive therapy for depression: A new approach to preventing relapse.* New York: Guilford.

Shalek, M. & Doyle, S. (1998). Relaxation revisited: An adaptation of a relaxation group geared toward geriatrics with behavior problems. *American Journal of Alzheimer's Disease and Other Dementias, 13*(3), 160–162.

Smith, A. (2004). Clinical uses of mindfulness training for older people. *Behavioral and Cognitive Psychotherapy, 32,* 423–430.

Smith, A. (2006). "Like waking up from a dream": Mindfulness training for older people with anxiety and depression. In R. A. Baer (Ed.), *Mindfulness-based treatment approaches* (pp. 191–212). Burlington, MA: Elsevier.

Tilden, V. P., Drach, L. L., & Tolle, S. W. (2004). Complementary and alternative therapy use at end-of-life in community settings. *The Journal of Alternative and Complementary Medicine, 10*(5), 811–817.

Toseland, R. W. (1995). *Group work with the elderly and family caregivers.* New York: Springer.

Wolff, I., van Croonenborg, J. J., Kemper, H.C.G., Kostense, P. J., & Twisk, J.W.R. (1999). The effect of exercise training programs on bone mass: A meta-analysis of published controlled trials in pre- and postmenopausal women. *Osteoporosis International, 9*(1), 1–12.

Wolsko, P.M., Eisenberg, D. M., Davis, R. B., & Phillips, R. S. (2004). Use of mind-body therapies: Results of a national survey. *Journal of General Internal Medicine, 19,* 43–50.

CHAPTER 5

Imagine This: Mindfulness-Based Elder Care for Frail Elders in the Nursing Home

IMAGINE THIS

Imagine walking into the dining/recreational area of a nursing home and seeing a group sitting silently in a circle. Their eyes may be open or closed, but they are very still. Some are in wheelchairs; most of the elders have obvious disabilities. The younger members are in uniforms, street clothes, or business attire. They are nursing home residents and staff, families, private aides, and volunteers. These definitions, however, are not relevant here. Right now, they are just people meditating together. Perhaps, there is aromatherapy, lavender, for example, in the room. Maybe even some quiet music. You know this is a nursing home, but it does not feel like one. It might even feel like a place you would want to be, a group you would want to be in.

OVERVIEW

Mindfulness classes in the nursing home can provide skills, support, and solace for residents and caregivers. This chapter describes the adaptations I made to the traditional model of mindfulness-based groups for a nursing home population. (See Chapter 2 for a description of Mindfulness-Based Stress Reduction and mindfulness-based groups.) These adaptations, which I have called Mindfulness-Based Elder Care, are based on experiences with a specific population, so further adaptations can be considered as needed. The key intention is to maintain the core integrity of this practice, and, at the same time, to adapt the presentation and teaching of the skills to enable a wide range of participants to benefit.

GROUP FORMAT

Traditionally, Mindfulness-Based Stress Reduction groups consist of 8 weeks of 2 1/2-hour classes, with the expectation of a daily homework practice, and 1 all-day session. I vary from this model in length, number, and expectations depending on the population and the environment. Group programs in the nursing home last 45 minutes to 1 hour. On a typical nursing home unit, there are residents with a variety of serious conditions and impairments, making longer groups impractical. I also find continuing groups to be more effective than time-limited groups. Nursing home residents face many challenges, and their skills may need ongoing reinforcement. All-day sessions are not offered.

For groups on the general nursing home unit, I limit resident inclusion to those who are able to follow simple instructions and are willing to try new techniques. Groups usually consist of 8 to 10 participants, all of whom self-identify as suffering from pain, stress, or both. It is easier to run groups if the attendees come consistently, but elders may be unable to attend regularly for a variety of reasons, including illness or medical appointments. For this reason, I usually open the groups to any residents who meet the above criteria, allowing members to join at any time. At times, unit staff sit in on a group. Groups are typically conducted in the dining area of the nursing home floors, since it is more easily accessible than other common areas. This choice facilitates participation by the maximum number of residents. These areas tend to be noisy, however, and frequent interruptions are likely. Sometimes, I use gentle music and aromatherapy to create a healing space. At other times, I encourage the group to be *present* with whatever distractions arise. Groups usually begin with a guided, quiet sitting. During this quiet sitting I encourage participants to pay attention to their breath, or their bodies, and to refocus their attention whenever their minds wander. Following this guided meditation, I check in with residents. Often, group members talk about new ways of responding to painful or stressful situations, describing how they have used techniques learned in previous groups to cope. Next, I introduce a new practice. New skills are learned by experience. Therefore, following the presentation, the members practice together, with time allowed for response and questions. The group ends with either guided imagery or silent meditation.

I find the Mindfulness-Based Elder Care (MBEC) groups in the nursing home to be a profound experience—for the residents and me. Group members quite powerfully express the anger and frustration of institutional life. They have lost not only much of their independence, but also their control over many aspects of their lives. My automatic inclination is to fix the pain, to offer a solution or advice. Sitting with my own discomfort is intense, but allows me to share in the experience of the residents. Following this discomfort, I often experience a deep sense of understanding and honor for this encounter.

SKILLS

Mindfulness teaches informal and formal skills that, if practiced regularly, may reduce suffering. These practices may also lead to profound life changes. For some, it is tempting to assume the skills without the deeper intent. The techniques, as noted earlier, are the "finger pointing at the moon," not the moon itself. Most important is the instructor's understanding and embodiment of the underlying principles of this practice. Below, I will share some adaptations of the skills for nursing home residents as well as recordings of group responses. More detailed descriptions of selected skills are given in Appendix A (yoga), B (guided meditations), and C (aromatherapy).

Mindful Eating

Mindfulness in daily living is frequently taught initially by an eating awareness. Engaging in a routine daily activity, in a slow attentive manner, often explains mindfulness in a way that words cannot. Group members are given a few raisins and asked to eat them slowly while observing their physical sensations, thoughts, and feelings. For many, eating is linked to nourishment at many levels. In nursing homes, food is very important. Eating can be an important activity in a resident's daily routine. In a culturally diverse nursing home, food preferences are quite varied. Some residents lose their sense of taste and may experience food differently. A bland or restricted diet may be medically indicated, but not preferred by the resident. As the facilitator of a Resident Council for many years, I was always struck by resident comments about the food. Some found the food too spicy, some not spicy enough. Some thought the vegetables were undercooked; some thought they were overcooked. I did not envy our dieticians. Given this relationship to food, a mindful eating experience is very helpful and very challenging.

> I passed around the raisins and asked the participants to hold them in their palms and describe them. Both Jose and Rose kept eating the raisins. I asked them again to pause and observe the raisins before eating them, and they did, briefly. I asked what happened. Jose said it felt "awful" to hold the raisins and wait to eat them. He said that

they have to wait for their food all the time. Anna said these raisins tasted better than any she had ever eaten.

The following week I asked if anyone had been able to practice eating mindfully. Many said that the dining room was noisy, and it was difficult to pay attention. Sarah said that the food tasted better when she ate slowly and paid attention.

These comments from a group for nursing home residents highlight the challenges faced everyday when living in an institutional environment: waiting for food, eating on the institutional schedule, the noisy and chaotic dining experience. Learning to eat mindfully, however, can offer a new relationship to the experience of eating as well as a new way of experiencing other routine events.

There may be residents who are not able, for a variety of reasons, to follow all of the mindful eating instructions. There may be residents with swallowing difficulties or medical conditions that would prohibit certain foods. To include as many residents as possible in the experience, consider different foods or consider using pureed or chopped foods.

Meditation

In the meditation practice, I begin by asking participants to focus on their breath. Breath observation is something available to everyone who can follow instructions. This meditation practice is also important for residents who may feel limited in other ways. Our residents often cannot participate in the body movement or other exercises. The overriding focus of MBEC is on what group participants *can* do. So, I often tell residents that anyone who is breathing can participate! Sitting in meditation with nursing home residents demonstrates many of the principles of mindfulness. Residents often experience that they are more than a sum of their parts; that they are whole just as they are right now; there is nothing that needs fixing; there is more that is right with them than there is wrong. It is an absolutely leveling experience to *be* with the residents, for them and me, without needing to fix or be fixed, to help or be helped.

We began with quiet sitting for 10 minutes. When we finished, Anna said it was amazing that the same chairs she sat in for meals felt more comfortable during the group. Everyone laughed. Mae said that she had many thoughts: First, the breathing, then about my earlier response to her questions and my feelings about her and her feelings about me. I said that was an interesting example of how the mind works; she described it so well. I asked if anyone else had noticed thoughts like these. All nodded and Mary [a nursing assistant] said that her mind was the same way. Sarah said that she wasn't really able to pay attention to her breath because her mind kept wandering.

I said that it didn't matter that her mind wandered, what mattered was that she kept coming back.

The next week, we started with a 15-minute quiet sitting. I noted that residents appeared more settled, less agitated as the weeks passed. When we finished, I asked how people were. Theresa said she noticed a tingling in her hand. I asked if this was something new, or perhaps always there and she just now noticed because she was paying attention to her body. She thought it might have been there before, but she didn't notice like Anna noticing the chairs being comfortable. We went around and people mostly said they felt good, but had difficulty identifying where in their body they felt it. They just said, "all over."

Diaphragmatic Breathing

Deep breathing can be difficult for nursing home residents with breathing problems. I use this exercise as an opportunity to talk about expanding our limits. Each of us is aware of our unique physical and emotional edges, the limits we feel we cannot trespass. Mindfulness classes encourage participants to explore these limits, to know when we can expand and explore them, and when we need to respect them. I use deep breathing as an example of how we can stretch a little further each day with regular practice.

We practiced deep, belly breathing, and I asked if they felt any different following this experience. Most said no, some said they were not sure, and others said yes. I asked the group to practice the deep breathing at various times during the day or night.

The following week I asked if people had practiced the deep breathing. Mae said she practiced once, at night, and it helped her go back to sleep. Gwen said that she had trouble breathing "right" ever since she had trouble learning to swim. Sarah said that she could not breathe deeply because her shoulders would move. I suggested there was no wrong or right way to breathe, what was important was to observe what was happening in our bodies right here and now. Some residents reported using the deep breathing to help cope with distressing situations.

Gentle Yoga

Gentle yoga provides an opportunity for nursing home residents to experience physical pleasure and abilities. It illustrates the principles of mindfulness in the body. Many of the participants have disabilities preventing them from joining in all of the stretches, but all can partake in some way. For example, when I ask them to stretch their arms, I say that those who cannot use one arm should stretch the arm that is available to them. If they cannot move their arms at all, I ask them to focus on their breathing and imagine they are stretching with us. Residents never express any distress that they cannot participate in the exercises; to the contrary, they feel good to be included. I verbally explain, then demonstrate the yoga exercises and also go to individual residents who are confused to provide hands-on assistance.

> We did some chair yoga appropriate for those in wheelchairs. They all participated and were able to notice sensations in their bodies. We discussed holding tension, how/why we do it, and how we can learn to listen to our bodies. Helen [a nursing assistant] said that when she came into the group she felt really tired, but now she felt energized.

Guided Imagery

Many residents respond to the use of imagery as a resource to address pain. Sometimes, an exercise as simple as breathing into the pain and gently releasing it with the out breath can offer relief. For nursing home residents, imagery of nature may be especially helpful since residents are often unable to visit previously healing places in nature.

Mindfulness teaches us to be with what is, accepting life as it presents itself. Guided imagery could be perceived as a way to escape life as it is, or it can provide a powerful metaphor to illuminate the process of shifting to a mindful awareness. Note, however, that there are times when imagery that we anticipate will be healing and relaxing can have the opposite effect. I find the image of a beach very relaxing. Once, I was working with a somewhat confused resident and used this image. He appeared upset and was able to communicate that he had had a traumatic near drowning experience in the past. It is especially important to be sensitive to nonverbal cues with residents who are unable to communicate verbally.

> I asked them to imagine a beach, how it looked, smelled, sounded, and felt on their skin. I then asked them to feel the sun on their skin and to direct the warm healing light to any part of their body that needed help. We allowed the light to flow all through us, and then just followed our breath. This lasted 15 minutes. Afterward, people appeared relaxed. Mae and Anna went to sleep. People said they were able to imagine the beach.

Body Scan

Nursing home residents often see their bodies through the lens of our ageist society. They see disability, wrinkles, and illness. The body scan neutralizes this self-view by encouraging participants to observe their bodies slowly, part by part, without judgment or criticism. Initially, residents say they do not feel anything. Often gentle probing reveals that they felt, but discounted, many sensations. Some find the body scan to be a chance to explore the parts of their bodies that are not in pain or problematic. Sometimes, I include an exercise in which residents tighten, then relax muscles, to increase body awareness and understand how we hold tension in our bodies. The body scan can offer an opportunity to be grateful for what still works! Many describe the experience as relaxing. There is an increased awareness of the body as a whole, more than a series of conditions and problems.

> After the body scan, most residents said they felt very good, that they were aware of parts of their bodies they had not thought of for a while. Sarah said she could really feel her toes for the first time in a long while! Mae said she did not feel anything, since she had a cold. I said that sometimes we think we don't feel anything, but that since she had a cold she might be feeling the sensations of a runny nose, cough, or congestion. She said, "Well, yes, but I don't like to think about that."

Standing and Walking Meditations

Walking meditation is another traditional mindfulness practice. Participants are asked to stand or walk with an awareness of physical sensations, feelings, and thoughts. In many of the groups, participants are in wheelchairs or walk with walkers or canes. I use standing and walking meditations when participants can tolerate the exercise, and generally, for short periods of time. Residents in wheelchairs or those using walkers or canes can participate using these devices. Elders also may hold a greater appreciation for these simple tasks that others take for granted.

> We did the standing and walking meditation. All of the residents in this group could stand and walk for a short period of time. Most were able to observe physical sensations while standing and walking. Jose said, "It was like concentrating in a different way."

Group Discussion

Group discussion with residents in the nursing home will have a natural focus on the very real and immediate pain and distress of medical conditions and institutional living. Institutional living can lead to learned disability. Residents may feel disempowered and unable to control any aspect of their lives, leaving it to "professionals." In the nursing home context, both residents and professionals identify with their roles of helper and helped. I remind residents that this group was not about fixing problems. In mindfulness groups, we discuss and learn new ways of being with pain and distress. Residents discover they are not frail victims, but participants and observers in their lives. Through MBEC groups, residents find that they still have abilities, control over their perceptions, and increased choices in how they respond to situations. Group discussion often starts with a resident complaining about having to wait for care provision or other residents or the food or pain. Rather than focus on resolving these issues, we use cognitive restructuring and discuss how what we practice and learn in the group might help with this particular situation. If a resident is upset because she had to wait to get a glass of water, for example, we might discuss what she could do while she waited. She could take a deep breath, practice meditation or stretches. Another simple exercise we discuss is S.T.O.P.

TRY THIS

S.T.O.P.! A Breathing Space

Stop, pause
Take a breath and Tune in. . . .
Observe what is happening in your body—notice physical sensations, thoughts, and feelings.
Proceed . . . with greater control and clarity.
Practice—patience—and persistence help, too!

This shift in focus enables residents to feel increased control over situations where previously they felt victimized and dependent.

Bess said that her roommate was still bothering her and that she would yell at her. We discussed the fight or flight response to stress. Group members discussed different stressful situations and how they responded. Ed, Mae, and Bess said they would fight. Theresa said when her roommate bothers her, she turns off her hearing aid. Rose says she doesn't listen. I said that sounded like a flight response. I encouraged residents to consider a third choice: mindfulness or using the skills we were practicing in this group. For example, when experiencing difficulty with a roommate, residents might consider becoming aware of their breathing and taking a moment to S. T. O. P.

Even in the nursing home, elders may feel isolated by communication barriers and fear of further loss. As one resident pointed out, "This is something I need because I spend a lot of solitary time." Mindfulness groups not only connect us to others in the group, but also may create a sense of connection to the larger whole beyond time and place.

Homework

Traditionally, MBSR group participants are asked to start a daily practice, using tapes, CDs, and other exercises assigned by the instructor. I found this type of homework to be impractical for nursing home residents due to their cognitive and physical challenges. In one of my first groups, I purchased cassette tape players and made tapes with a guided body scan for the participants. The residents unanimously did not utilize the tapes. The residents were unfamiliar with these small devices and uncomfortable with learning how to use them. Although my experience of using cassette players with this group was not successful, I have found the use of tapes to be very successful in two other circumstances: both with the Telephone Wellness Group and with responsive individuals who were aided by staff. These circumstances will be discussed in Chapters 6 and 7.

> I asked about the homework. Theresa said that she fell asleep whenever she lay down. Mae said that she had been sick. Everyone is having difficulty with the tape players. I said I could come around tomorrow and help out. I said that if the tape players were difficult, they could just do the breathing exercises.

Traditional mindfulness-based group homework assignments include introducing regular meditation and yoga practices into a daily routine, recording pleasant and unpleasant events, and practicing mindfulness in daily life. I find these longer assignments challenging in the nursing home because the residents often do not remember these practices. On the other hand, I do find the residents use the deep breathing practice a lot and report that it helps them in dealing with the overriding loss of control they experience in the nursing home. Residents also regularly report that they are better able to cope with the stresses of nursing home life by using the skills practiced during group.

Pleasant and Unpleasant Experiences

Mindfulness-based classes often include a homework assignment that asks participants to record a daily log of pleasant experiences throughout the week. Participants are asked to observe the experience, their feelings, thoughts, and physical sensations in the moment. The following week, participants are asked to track unpleasant experiences and observe their feelings, thoughts, and physical sensations related to these moments. In my early groups, I realized that physical and cognitive limitations might prevent residents from recording their experiences over the week, so I adapted the practice to a discussion within the group.

I talked about the connection between our mind and our body. The residents looked a little blank. I realized that these group members would probably not be able to fill out the pleasant/unpleasant experiences chart as a homework assignment. I suggested that everyone think of something that they really enjoyed—perhaps, ice cream, their grandchildren, a trip. We closed our eyes and thought about this experience for a few moments and also about any physical sensations we might be having while thinking about this experience. I asked people to report back. Everyone in the group was able to experience a pleasant event and also stated that they felt physical sensations associated with it. Some said they felt warm. Others said they felt the experience in their heart.

Following this discussion, I asked members to think about an unpleasant experience and any physical sensations associated with it. Members also reported experiences and sensations of discomfort. Helen said she just wanted to get away. Others felt stomach discomfort. Others felt nervous. After this, I was able to point out the mind-body connection again, and the residents really responded this time!

Lovingkindness Meditation

As discussed in the previous section, lovingkindness, compassion, and forgiveness are key components of mindfulness practice. For elders facing disability, loss, and death, forgiveness and compassion practice can offer resolution and spiritual support. At times, group members reported a connection to their spiritual roots.

> One group member shared that during a meditation, she remembered the feeling she had as a young woman when lighting the candles for Shabbat dinner. A resident said, "This is good, it reminds me of a prayer." Another said, "This group makes me feel at peace with the world, it helps my whole body and spirit."

CONSIDERATIONS: ENVIRONMENTAL

Transportation

How easy is it for your residents to get to the group? In larger facilities, it may be difficult to gather residents for a group. They may be physically unable to get there, or they may get lost or forget the time and place. One solution is to limit the group to those who can physically get there and those who might only need one reminder. The location of the group is also a consideration. If the group is in a central location in the facility, it will allow access by more residents. On the other hand, groups offered on a unit that has the most need could make it easier for more of the residents to get there. I tried both and found it more manageable for me to run groups on the units and that more residents could benefit.

Group Space

The ideal space for a group is one that is easily accessible and quiet. Most nursing homes, however, lack accessible and quiet spaces. They are often noisy and have a distinct scent. While newer models of providing care seek to create a more homelike environment, few facilities have completed this transition and few have quiet, accessible space appropriate for running groups. Mindfulness practice teaches us to be with what is rather than wanting things to be different. And yet, learning the new skills of stress reduction in a common area where there are constant interruptions may be difficult, especially for nursing home residents also facing multiple personal problems. While it may seem contradictory to the basic tenet of letting things be as they are, in challenging environments it can be helpful to use aids to establish a sense of healing space. At the same time, participants can be encouraged to practice independently in any environment.

The MBEC groups that I run are in the dining room on a nursing home unit. The chairs are set in a circle at one end of the room, and if there are screens or partitions, I use them. For most groups on the nursing home units, I use classical or other quiet music and aromatherapy to create a protected space in which residents can nurture the skills they are learning. If possible, the lights can be dimmed. At other times, the group practice is to *be* with whatever comes up. Residents and staff often found the aromatherapy to be an especially significant part of their experience.

CONSIDERATIONS: POPULATION

Group Inclusion Criteria: Cognitive Status

In a mixed group setting, it is important to consider the benefits of including many residents versus the challenges of including residents with cognitive decline. Residents with mild dementia will still be able to follow instructions and participate. They also can really gain from the group as a place to focus on their inner strengths and abilities. Residents with moderate dementia will need to be assessed individually for the appropriateness of inclusion. While most residents will be able to benefit from the group, disruptive behaviors will impact the environment for other group members. Residents with severe cognitive challenges may be better suited for their own group, modeled on the group I will discuss in the following chapter.

You may find some residents are disruptive at times either by being verbally or physically agitated. In my groups, it is not uncommon for a group member to begin talking in the midst of a meditation. When this happens, I either address their question or concern, or ask the resident if he or she can wait until the meditation or other exercise is finished. Most important, I consider how I address the resident as a message to that resident and to the other group members. I want the entire group to be able to continue their practice, but I also consider if I am rigidly insisting on my agenda rather than remaining open to the individuals in the group.

> While we were sitting in quiet meditation, Sarah got up and said she was cold. We helped her move, and I made sure the windows were shut. Then, after a few minutes, Sarah said, "What is the name of this group anyway?" Other residents began opening their eyes curiously. I asked if she could wait until we finished the meditation. I said there would be time later for questions. When we finished, Mae said she was hot, and I helped her take off her sweater.

ENDINGS

A key component of many mindfulness-based groups is that they are time-limited. For nursing home residents, however, I find that ongoing groups are more beneficial. Carryover, the ability to maintain the practices and learning, may be difficult due to cognitive deficits. As one resident said, "When I go back to my room, I will think about what we did in the group, but I'll forget it by tomorrow."

In addition, residents face multiple daily challenges in the nursing home, and ongoing reinforcement of the skills and group support is especially helpful here. As previously discussed, residents did utilize some of the practices like deep breathing and cognitive restructuring, but needed frequent reminders to practice other skills outside of class. Concrete aids, including handouts and the exercise described below, can also help participants recall the mindfulness practices. I generally run ongoing groups, but the following discussion illustrates residents' response to the ending of a time-limited group.

LAST GROUP

We opened the discussion with how things were going, how members were feeling. Everyone kept asking if this was really the last class. I said it was. We talked about what people had gotten from the class, and most said breathing. We practiced the meditation we had learned of following our breath for 20 minutes. As we ended, I asked members to consider what they had found personally helpful in our group—a word or thought from their present experience that they would like to keep with them.

As we ended the meditation, I asked the group to hold the thought or word. I gave them each cards and asked them to write the phrase on the card. When they finished, I asked them to take the cards with them to use later to remind them of what was helpful.

MEASURING RESULTS: MBEC RESEARCH

My impressions, based on observations and reports from attendees, consistently found the MBEC groups to be helpful. But how did they help? Was any of it measurable? While quality of life is considered as essential as quantity, it is more difficult to measure. It is especially difficult to measure with nursing home residents (Gerritsen, Steverink, Ooms, de Vet, & Ribbe, 2007; Kane, 2003). In addition, this cohort is not skilled at emotional expression and may become even less skilled as cognition diminishes. Qualitative reports from elders tend to be simple and concrete: "I feel better." "This is good."

Initially, I administered, or attempted to administer, research tools to identify the residents' cognitive status, depression, pain, and stress level pre- and post- an 8-week group for 10 residents. Results were inconclusive due to a poor completion rate and did not demonstrate the effect I witnessed and that residents reported. I was especially struck by the lack of carryover in effect given what I anecdotally noted from the verbal and nonverbal responses of participants. I knew that after the groups, residents would report feeling more relaxed and able to cope. In the groups, they also reported that they were using the practices to help with stressful circumstances outside the group. These results suggest that ongoing short groups, without homework assignments, are the most beneficial for the nursing home resident.

In 2002, I followed one MBEC group for 10 weeks. Inclusion criteria were minimal—an ability to follow simple instructions and an openness to trying new techniques. Groups usually consisted of 8 to 10 participants, all of whom were referred by staff or had identified themselves as suffering from pain, stress, or both. The group utilized the MBEC model discussed above. Each group was treated as a single session, and residents were assessed pre- and postgroup. Two questions from the Coop Inventory on pain and general life satisfaction were used. The feelings scale is a 1 to 5 visual analogue scale with a score of 1 indicating having no pain and 5 indicating having severe pain (Nelson, Landgraf, Hays, Wasson, & Kirk, 1990). Posttest, residents were also asked if they felt any different after spending 1 hour in the program and, if so, to describe the difference. Statistical analysis included frequency distributions and nonparametric statistical tests for continuous variables.

These findings were more conclusive (McBee, Westreich, & Likourezos, 2004). We measured the participants for pain and general well-being. Results showed that after the group, members reported feeling less sad ($p <$ 0.001), and a trend toward feeling less pain ($p = 0.094$). This is consistent with mindfulness tenets: while we cannot change what is, we can change how we view it. In qualitative reports, residents clearly expressed the impact of the group. Many, when asked to describe how they felt, stated simply: "I like this group" and "I learned something." The most frequently reported benefit of these groups is the sense of connection with others. The following are other quotes from residents about the group:

> I feel uplifted. I realize we all have pain. We talk about how we are getting along. It is important to be with other people.
> I've always liked this [group] since I started . . . being quiet, relaxed . . . a special feeling.
> I enjoy being with people and talking. We all have our own problems and can help each other.

As former Surgeon General Jocelyn Elders (1994) once pointed out, health care (including preventative health care) is only effective when it is accessible. For elders with loss and disability, the benefits of mindfulness can offer empowerment, as well as a sense of wholeness and connection. In order to convey the principles of mindfulness, the skills can be adapted and presented in ways that make them accessible to this population.

REFERENCES

Elders, J. (1994, May). Commencement speech at the Columbia School of Public Health Graduation, New York.

Gerritsen, D. L., Steverink, N., Ooms, M. E., de Vet, H.C.W., & Ribbe, M. W. (2007). Measurement of overall quality of life in nursing homes through self-report: The role of cognitive impairment. *Quality of Life Research, 16*(6), 1029–1037.

Kane, R. A. (2003). Definition, measurement, and correlates of quality of life in nursing homes: Toward a reasonable practice, research, and policy agenda. *The Gerontologist, 43,* 28–36.

McBee, L., Westreich, L., & Likourezos, A. (2004). A psychoeducational relaxation group for pain and stress management in the nursing home. *Journal of Social Work in Long-Term Care, 3*(1), 15–28.

Nelson, E. C., Landgraf, J. M., Hays, R. D., Wasson, J. H., & Kirk, J. W. (1990, December). The functional status of patients: How can it be measured in physicians' offices? *Medical Care, 28*(12), 1111–1126.

CHAPTER 6

Drifting Away From My Head
to My Heart: Mindfulness-Based
Elder Care for Elders
With Dementia

*I race up and down the corridors of my mind, frantically seeking to make
sense of what's going on around me. Sometimes this process makes me even
more lost, and I become lost about why I am lost. (Taylor, 2007, p. 35)*

Understanding and providing care and support for persons with dementia
requires great compassion and skill on the part of the caregiver. Self-care and a
personal mindfulness practice are often good starting points. In addition, conveying mindfulness via groups and individual interventions for persons with
dementia may offer relief from the distress and fear that often accompanies this
condition. Adjustments to the model are necessary, even though persons with
dementia are in some ways more open to the concept of mindfulness or being
in the present moment. The interventions described below are, more than
ever, solely guidelines. I describe a mindfulness-based group, as well as other
interventions that are not specific to mindfulness, but that can be implemented
mindfully. The most important intervention is our authentic presence in each
interaction. Caring for this population requires openness, flexibility, creativity,
and an ability to work from the heart. It is also helpful to remember that we all
have the basic needs to be valued, to communicate, and to connect.

WHAT DO WE KNOW ABOUT DEMENTIA?

I think, therefore I exist.

—Descartes

The inner space of our brains remains mysterious while the number of persons impacted by dementia increases. International studies document that 1 in 20 people over the age of 65 suffer from diseases causing dementia and 1 in 5 of those over the age of 80. An estimated 24 million people live with dementia worldwide. It is predicted that this number will rise to 81 million by 2040 (Alzheimer's Disease International, n.d.). The estimated cost of dementia care is currently $315 billion annually worldwide (Wimo, Winblada, & Jonssonb, 2007). The direct cost of dementia care in the United States, where numbers diagnosed with Alzheimer's doubled from 1980 to 2000, is highest, estimated in 2005 at $76 billion (Hebert, Scherr, Bienias, Bennett, & Evans, 2003; Wimo et al., 2007). Long-term costs, including caregiver's missed work and stress-related illness, could add significantly to this price tag.

Alzheimer's disease, multi-infarct or vascular dementia, Pick's disease, Parkinson's disease, Creutzfeldt–Jakob disease, Huntington's disease, and Lewy body syndrome are considered the primary categories of dementia. Dementia is generally not cured, but instead, can only be managed or its progress slowed. As with cancer and AIDS, we may increasingly find ways to live with dementia and to modify its impact through environmental and behavioral interventions. Pioneers of current behavioral interventions advocate offering emotional support rather than information, correction, and reality orientation. Feil's *Validation Breakthrough* (2002) and Bell and Troxel's *Best Friend's Approach to Alzheimer's Care* (2003) both focus on positive engagement, reinforcing the strengths of the person with dementia.

In addition to books by professionals, persons diagnosed with Alzheimer's disease have written several recent books. Authors such as Robert Taylor (2007), Diana Friel McGowin (1993), and Thomas DeBaggio (2002) offer a personal and profound insight into the process of the disease. These authors clearly describe their confusion and angst. At the same time, they consistently remind readers that, while they become increasingly confused, they experience the same feelings as all of us. In fact, feelings appear to take precedence over thoughts. Dr. Taylor describes it as "drifting away from my head and into my heart" (p. 128). Social skills may remain, without comprehension of the meaning of these skills. Need for autonomy and control remain. McGowin, in *Living in the Labyrinth,* describes the isolation and despair of Alzheimer's:

> Each one of us must feel they have worth as a living being. . . . I feel my lack of worth acutely when I am in large groups of people. . . . Painfully lonely, I still contrarily, deliberately, sit alone in my home. . . . Somewhere there is that ever-present reminder list of what I am supposed to do today. But I cannot find it. (1993, p. 112)

When relating to persons with dementia, seeing the whole person, not just the disease, is fundamental.

COMMUNICATION WITH PERSONS WITH DEMENTIA

Communicating with persons with dementia is challenging, exciting, frightening, and frustrating. It takes courage and creativity, trial and error, and a willingness to be one's authentic self. As a social work instructor for student interns, I assigned each student to a person with advanced dementia. It enabled the students to learn ways and to interact from the heart rather than the head. A fellow teacher and friend describes how he prepares to teach people with dementia: "You enter a space with people that are in that way of being in the world, and work from there." He also discusses how assumptions about what and who are benefiting from the teaching can be misleading. Group members may not appear to be responding to the exercises, and then, will lift an arm or leg, or smile. It is important to assume that mindfulness practices are still being communicated despite a lack of clear or usual response (L. Sierra, personal communication, August 10, 2007).

Following are basic tips on communication adapted in part from the Alzheimer's Association (n.d.):

- Center yourself and focus fully on the person with whom you are communicating.
- Consider your tone, pace, body language, and other nonverbal cues.
- Maintain eye contact and use simple, concrete language.
- Provide instructions that are one step at a time.
- Minimize environmental distractions.
- Try not to correct the person with dementia.
- Use touch to reinforce, but also consider that for some touch is not welcome.
- Allow time to respond.
- Listen to verbal and nonverbal communication.
- Accept persons as they are.
- Connect with and respond to the feeling of what is being expressed.

Many of these communication principles reflect a mindful interaction: paying attention to the moment, nonjudgmentally; engaging the whole self; tuning in to the environment; becoming acutely aware of our impact on others. At the same time we consider our own affect, it is helpful to read the affect of the person with dementia. If words cannot be understood, perhaps facial expressions can. Happiness, fear, and sadness may all be communicated and commented on. It is important to ask the person to verify the emotion rather than to assume it, however. Listening mindfully is especially helpful here. Many who work with this population have been startled by moments of clarity expressed by persons who seem profoundly demented. One woman, diagnosed with end-stage dementia and nonverbal, slid from her chair one day. The nurse, who always spoke to her despite the lack of response, asked if she was all right. The woman responded, "Yes, thank you." When working with this population, it is always important to assume that they understand everything.

In addition, verbal responses from this population initially may not make sense, but when carefully listened to, almost like poetry or a mystery, can offer clues to meaning. In one group on a dementia unit, one of the members died. The other group members did not specifically comment on her absence but asked later about the "baby on the bicycle." This was a confusing statement until the group leaders remembered that the resident who died was very petit, often stuck out her tongue repeatedly, and was in a wheelchair (Bober, McClellan, McBee, & Westreich, 2002). Nonverbal communication can also offer connections. Using the senses, including those of smell, touch, and taste, provides stimulation and reminiscence. Aromatherapy, for example, can evoke strong memories and emotions for some.

Elders with dementia usually suffer from other physical conditions and communication limitations. Take into consideration vision or hearing impairments as well as other conditions that impact communication.

HELEN

Helen was taken to the emergency room after a fall at home. The ER staff observed that she was confused and nonsensical, unable to understand their questions. She became frustrated and agitated, and the ER staff gave her medications and restrained her, diagnosing her with dementia. When her community social worker finally came to the ER, she informed hospital xstaff that Helen's hearing aids were left at home during the hospital transport. She was not demented; she could not hear.

BEHAVIORS ACCOMPANYING DEMENTIA

All behavior is an attempt to communicate. Elders with dementia possess the same basic needs we all do: the need to feel connected and valued, the need to communicate and to be stimulated. When other avenues of communication are lost, behavior, and at times aggressive behavior, can be the only avenue of communication.

SIMON

Simon, a 79-year-old widower, was admitted to a dementia unit. This particular unit was for residents with dementia and challenging behavior. Simon's behavior was the most difficult when bath time arrived. He required five people to take him to the bath, one for each extremity. And still, he would spit at those who held him down. His screams wracked the entire unit. When the psychiatrist was consulted, she noted that Simon was a Holocaust survivor and suggested that the bath would recreate the trauma of that experience. When staff began to give Simon a sponge bath in his room, there was no longer any behavior problem with bathing.

Books by persons with dementia describe their distress. Persons with dementia who are no longer able to express feelings verbally often evidence physical agitation or difficult behaviors. Disrobing, hitting, wandering, calling out all may be attempts to communicate a specific need, or a general cry of distress. Stress reduction skills can offer relief and repose to agitated persons in a nonjudgmental format.

GROUP LEADER

TRY THIS: NONVERBAL COMMUNICATION

As you interact with others, note the nonverbal communications you are receiving and sending. Notice body language. Hear the tone, cadence, rhythm, and intensity of speech. Observe facial expressions. What would you "hear" if you did not understand the words?

A key element in MBEC groups and interactions is a personal mindfulness practice. When I am centered and calm, even residents who cannot follow instructions or respond cognitively to the techniques are able to respond positively to mindfulness interventions. While some might not understand the guided imagery or instructions, all can respond to the tone of my voice, my body language, and an environment of acceptance and healing.

Perhaps we may avoid communication with elders with dementia because it calls for effort, great creativity, patience, and an ability to use verbal and nonverbal skills. Attempting to communicate with persons with dementia may take us out of our comfort zone as the professional who knows everything. We must be willing to individualize treatment, use trial and error, tolerate feelings of helplessness and confusion, and vulnerability. And we must take responsibility for communication, not merely blame the demented person. Or perhaps we are afraid:

I believe Alzheimer's has replaced cancer as the most feared disease people can imagine. (Taylor, 2007, p. 51)

If Alzheimer's is the most feared disease, what are the implications for professionals? Our first job is to examine our feelings about dementia and the persons who have it. Nowhere is it more important to know that our patients and we are the same and connected. Nowhere is it more challenging since we often define ourselves by the very abilities that persons with dementia lose. What does the philosophy of Descartes, "I think, therefore I exist," imply for a person with dementia? As they lose their cognition, are they not?

MBEC GROUPS

Superficially, it might appear that mindfulness-based groups should be restricted to participants who have a fair attention span and are able to follow instructions. Mindfulness practice by nursing home residents with behavioral problems and moderate to severe dementia demonstrates, however, that these practices transcend the residents' cognitive conditions. On a special care unit for such residents, a psychiatrist and I co-led an ongoing mindfulness-based group for 18 months. The group, consisting of 5 to 10 residents, followed a simple structure: deep breathing and some gentle stretches, discussion, if appropriate, and guided imagery to end the group. Aromatherapy and music helped create a sacred space in the midst of a noisy hospital dining room where confused residents often wandered in and out. If a resident were extremely agitated and disruptive, we would attempt to calm him or her by one-to-one interaction and gentle touch. Often physical agitation could be incorporated into the group. For example, if a resident could not sit still, we might walk with that resident mindfully (Lantz, Buchalter, & McBee, 1997).

In a current group, I have broken away from the original structured format. In preparation, I gauge the participants' energy level. If I sense the group is agitated and overwhelmed, I will put on lavender aromatherapy and calming music and do breathing exercises and gentle stretches. On the other hand, if I sense the group is tired and lethargic, I will use peppermint oil and salsa, or other energizing music, to stretch or dance to. I often hand out simple musical instruments, and we all play along to the music. Sometimes, I encourage the group to be noisy—sighing or verbalizing with stretches, or humming. I will start a laughter meditation this way, encouraging participants to laugh out loud. Initially forced, it usually results in a good belly laugh. Laughter is something we can all share! With this group, I often end with a gentle shoulder rub for residents, which most enjoy.

Seated Meditation

Some may believe that persons with moderate to advanced dementia are not capable of quiet, seated meditation. While residents engaged in my groups may have periods of agitation, many also are able to quiet down, follow simple instructions, or, at least, respond to a calming environment. Using visual cues, responding to outbursts with acceptance and redirection, often settles down the group. I find the most important intervention is my intention to connect in the group, staying with this intention despite frequent distractions.

COMPLEMENTARY AND ALTERNATIVE INTERVENTIONS ON A DEMENTIA UNIT

As previously discussed, connecting to persons with dementia requires multi-faceted and creative approaches that are often nonverbal. Other interventions that are not specific to mindfulness practice but can connect nonverbally with elders are aromatherapy, breathing exercises, simple stretches, hand massage, and guided imagery.

Breathing Exercises

Breathing exercises offer persons with dementia a stress reduction activity that can be easily understood and accomplished. In demonstrating breathing exercises, I use visual cues as well as verbal. Placing my hands on my belly, I demonstrate diaphragmatic breathing. I then place my hands on my ribs, and finally, on my upper chest. Persons with dementia often perform exercises in a copycat fashion, as they attempt to follow and understand. I have even noted that when I scratch my nose, the residents will follow my visual, rather than verbal, instructions, even where not appropriate! During these exercises, I also may approach individual participants and guide their hands to their belly, ribs, or upper chest. Sometimes, I hold a seated resident's two hands and gently lift them up as I invite her to breathe in, and I lower the hands as I cue her to breathe out. Many elders sit folded over in their chairs, and gently lifting their arms overhead allows for more breathing space in the torso. Breathing exercises can be done in combination with imagery. I may ask group members to breathe in, using their arms to gather up all the things they want in their life and to breathe out as they use their arms to push away what they don't want: pain, stress, anger. Most important, I offer lots of encouragement and positive feedback.

Aromatherapy

The addition of aromatherapy to a dementia unit can provide a simple, cost-effective intervention that benefits both those who receive care and those who give it. Supplies are easily available and Appendices C and F provide more information. I use aromatherapy diffusers in groups, and also use individual applications, administering the oils via cotton balls and waving under the resident's nose. I also provide the oils on cotton balls for staff, for their own use and for use later with the residents. In addition, I combine essential oils with carrier oils for massage (see below).

Hand Massage

Hand massage can be utilized individually or in a group setting. Persons with dementia may be unused to, or even frightened, by touch. I find that approaching residents carefully, sitting at eye level, making eye contact, and asking permission, is a good way to introduce hand massage. If the person does not seem to understand my words, I will hold their hand gently and demonstrate briefly, using nonverbal cues. I also observe for nonverbal negative reactions. Persons with dementia generally enjoy this intervention. The soft, gentle, repetitive stroking is noninvasive and connects the massage giver and massage receiver through touch, at times, the only remaining avenue of communication available. I usually begin by using almond oil mixed with an essential oil. I have found that some people really like the way the oil makes their skin soft. Some do not, however, and the hand massage can be administered without oils with good effect. I often note tension and holding in the hands I am massaging and relaxation following the massage. For elders whose hands are contracted or arthritic, this massage can offer relief when done gently. (See Appendix C for a more detailed description.)

Guided Imagery

Using guided imagery, especially verbally, may seem inappropriate for persons with moderate to severe dementia. I have found that many in this population will benefit from guided imagery with simple accommodations. Awareness of nonverbal communication is especially important here. Facial expression, eye contact, body language, and tone of voice all convey meaning. Persons with dementia can be especially sensitive to unspoken affect and emotion, and the practitioner's demeanor may speak louder than his or her words. For the practitioner, then, grounding in mindfulness practice is key. In addition, using simple, concrete language and repetition can assist persons with cognitive deficits to understand the imagery. I also use environmental cues. For example, when using ocean imagery in a group, I give participants sea-shells or beach stones to hold, and I use ocean sounds. Often residents who appear unable to understand verbal interaction respond to this imagery. One such resident stated that he remembered going to the beach, and he smiled. Again, with this population, the responses may be limited and unclear, so it is important to watch for nonverbal cues, either positive or not, in gauging the response to guided imagery.

Yoga Stretches

Persons with dementia often evidence physical agitation, such as restless walk-ing or banging on a table. In some environments, their movements may be restricted for safety. This may add to their distress and decline in functioning. In groups, I always include stretches. The general principles I employ are to use chair stretches and to stretch in all directions. For example, I include a stretch up to the ceiling, even when seated, verbally encouraging participants to stretch their entire body: fingers, hands, arms, shoulders, chest and torso, hips, legs and feet. I then may ask participants to fold over, gently, in an inver-sion, resting their folded arms on their laps or the table. We also twist from side to side in the chair, looking over each shoulder. Extra movements of the hands and feet, rotating the joints and shaking them out can be fun and releasing. I make sure to observe the participants so that they do not surpass their limits.

More recently, I have been combining reminiscence, guided imagery, and exercise. When describing exercises, I will use imagery that relates to a famil-iar activity. For example, when teaching finger movement exercises, I will ask participants to "play the piano," or when teaching scalp self-massage, I will ask participants to "shampoo their hair." Another familiar movement I have used is rocking a baby. Chapter 8 has a list of many of the movements I have used. I also combine longer guided imageries with movement. For example, when using a beach-guided imagery, I ask participants to go into the water and swim, demonstrating different arm strokes and breathing. Or, we will go for a "walk" as we move our feet up and down while seated.

A GROUP EXERCISE USING IMAGERY AND MOVEMENT

We went for a walk, and I asked them where they would like to go. Eleanor said, "Times Square," Frank said the forest, and John said the beach. I asked if it was all right to choose the forest today, and they said yes and smiled. We moved our feet up and down, sometimes faster, sometimes slower. We also swung our arms as we "walked." I suggested what we might experience in the forest: the sound of trees and birds, the smell of flowers, the air on our skin. They were all smiling and moving their feet up and down. Sally said what about the mosquitoes? So we imagined a breeze that would blow them away. Some laughed at this. They all seemed to thoroughly engage in this exercise. We used all of our senses—sight, smell, sound, touch, taste.

Another movement that this group seems to enjoy is the self-hug! I combine this with a breathing exercise, asking them to open their arms wide as they breathe in and hug themselves as they breathe out. I have used the image of a flower opening and closing when I could bring in flowers. They often giggle and smile. Movement to music can inspire the group leader as well as participants and is discussed in Chapter 8. For group leaders, these movements provide an opportunity to connect with their inner child and to have fun—and having fun is contagious!

THE FLORENCE V. BURDEN STUDY ON THE DEMENTIA UNIT

A grant was awarded to the nursing home by the Florence V. Burden Foundation to incorporate four Complementary and Alternative (CAM) interventions into the care plans on a special care unit for residents with dementia and behavioral problems. The expectation was that these interventions—aromatherapy, breathing exercises, hand massage, and guided imagery—would improve quality of life, relieve pain, and reduce behavioral difficulties. All staff on the experimental unit, including evening and night, were trained in the modalities, and a CAM Trainer was on the unit 10 hours a week. CAM modalities were included in individual care planning for the residents based on their needs, conditions, and responses. On a control unit, identical in size and patient and staff composition, care was provided without the addition of CAM. Results were measured for one year, using the Cohen-Mansfield Agitation Inventory (Koss et al., 1997) and the Cornell Scale for Depression in Dementia (Alexopoulos, Abrams, Young, & Shamoian, 1988). Both scales use staff reports; in this case, nurses and nursing assistants were interviewed. Unpublished findings demonstrated statistically significant decline in both agitation ($p < 0.01$) and depression ($p < 0.05$).

Anecdotal findings also testify to the effectiveness of CAM modalities with these confused and agitated elders. Nonverbal elders responded to hand massages with sighs, slower breathing, and visible muscle release. Aromatherapy was very popular with both staff and residents. One resident, who was losing weight, began to eat more and gained three pounds when cinnamon essential oil was utilized prior to mealtime. A few drops of lavender essential oil in the bath helped calm residents who became agitated at bath time. Below are three case studies written by the CAM Trainer:

BESS

Bess sits hunched in a chair with her head in her lap for most of the day. Initially, I thought there would be little I could do with her to help. But when I wave a cotton ball with peppermint oil under her nose, Bess invariably awakes, opens her eyes, lifts her head, and looks right at you. Often, this is accompanied with a smile and even a laugh. Once she's awake, I am able to give her hand massages and do gentle arm stretches with her that we coordinate with our breath. These therapies usually leave her awake and sitting in a better posture, so that she can breathe more easily. There have even been a few times where Bess has tried to say something to me, but the words didn't come out right. Bess is a good example of how we never know just exactly how someone is going to react to these therapies.

RALPH

Ralph loves the breathing and guided imagery tapes and really responds to the aromatherapy as well. Still able to cognitively process many things, Ralph can be provocative and often gets himself into altercations with other residents. The CAM therapies have really improved that behavior. These therapies can keep him engaged for hours and help prevent negative interactions with other residents. The other way in which the therapies have helped Ralph is at bath time. He used to be extremely combative at bath time, and now with a little lavender in the bath water and the playing of a guided imagery tape during bath time, he is much more cooperative. It's really changed the experience for him as well as the staff.

STELLA

Stella is bed-ridden, does not communicate, and is fed through a feeding tube. Direct verbal interaction was out of the question. I decided to try hand massages with her. Touch seems to calm her down, stop her hands from shaking, and let her know that someone is in the room with her. Invariably, her breathing seems to slow down when I give her a hand massage, as if she senses our interaction and is comforted by it. This is also a good example of how we can "listen" to nonverbal residents by observing their breath (Lombardo, McBee, Lantz, & Cronin, 2004).

While aromatherapy, hand massage, guided imagery, and breathing exercises may not change the course of disease and dementia, they may moderate behavior and improve day-to-day quality of life for distressed and confused elders.

MBEC not only provides comfort to the group members but also demonstrates new capacities in these residents by staff and caregivers. In the 1996 Wellness Group, staff perceived a reduction in agitation and behavioral problems on the unit (Lantz et al., 1997). For me, this group created a new connection with confused residents. When we identify our selfhood with our minds, the loss of memory can represent the loss of self. In mindfulness practice, we experience a realm more profound than the mind. From this realm, we experience the interconnection of all beings.

REFERENCES

Alexopoulos, G. S., Abrams, R. C., Young, R. C., & Shamoian, C. A. (1988). Depression in dementia. *Biological Psychiatry, 1*(23), 271–284.

Alzheimer's Association. (n.d.) *Tips for better communication.* Retrieved July 28, 2007, from http://www.alz.org/living_with_alzheimers_communication.asp

Alzheimer's Disease International. (n.d.). *The global impact of dementia.* Retrieved July 28, 2007, from http://www.alz.co.uk/media/dementia.html

Bell, V., & Troxel, D. (2003). *The best friend's approach to Alzheimer's care.* Baltimore: Health Professionals.

Bober, S., McClellan, E., McBee, L., & Westreich, L. (2002). The Feelings Art Group: A vehicle for personal expression in skilled nursing home residents with dementia. *Journal of Social Work in Long-Term Care, 1*(4), 73–87.

DeBaggio, T. (2002). *Losing my mind: An intimate look at life with Alzheimer's.* New York: Free Press.

Feil, N. (2002). *The validation breakthrough* (2nd ed.). Baltimore: Health Professionals.

Hebert, L. E., Scherr, P. A., Bienias, J. L., Bennett, D. A., & Evans, D. A. (2003). Alzheimer disease in the U.S. population: Prevalence estimates using the 2000 census. *Archives of Neurology, 60*(8), 1119–1122.

Koss, E., Weiner, M., Ernesto, C., Cohen-Mansfield, J., Ferris, S. H., Grundman, M., et al. (1997). Assessing patterns of agitation in Alzheimer's disease patients with the Cohen-Mansfield Agitation Inventory. The Alzheimer's Disease Cooperative Study. *Alzheimer's Disease and Associated Disorders, 11*(Suppl. 2), S45–50.

Lantz, M. S., Buchalter, E., & McBee, L. (1997). The Wellness Group: A novel intervention for coping with disruptive behavior in elderly nursing home residents. *The Gerontologist, 37*(4), 551–556.

Lombardo, A., McBee, L., Lantz, M. L., & Cronin, D. (2004). *Complementary Alternative Medicine manual for nursing homes: Findings and insights from a project at the Jewish Home and Hospital.* Unpublished manual.

McGowin, D. F. (1993). *Living in the labyrinth.* New York: Dell.

Taylor, R. (2007). *Alzheimer's from the inside out.* Baltimore: Health Professionals.

Wimo, A., Winblada, B., & Jonssonb, L. (2007). An estimate of the total worldwide societal costs of dementia in 2005. *Alzheimer's & Dementia: The Journal of the Alzheimer's Association, 3*(2), 81–91.

CHAPTER 7

Got to Go Through the Door: Mindfulness-Based Elder Care for Isolated Elders and Palliative Care

So high, can't get over it
So low, can't go under it
So wide, can't get around it
Got to go through the door.

—Traditional camp song

Bill Thomas cites the three plagues of institutionalized frail elders as loneliness, helplessness, and boredom (Thomas, 2004). These plagues may also apply to isolated homebound elders. This chapter discusses working one to one with elders who are isolated, whether in the nursing home or homebound, and those at the end of life. For both formal and informal caregivers, the greatest challenge may be working with their own feelings about illness and death. Here, mindfulness practice can guide those who give care and those who receive it.

Elders are increasingly isolated for many reasons. They may be home or bed bound by chronic ailments that affect their mobility. They may be hard of hearing, confused; they may forget words or be unable to speak. Elders may be separated from family and friends due to loss, distance, conflicting responsibilities, or relationships. Professional caregivers involved with elders are increasingly rewarded for completing paperwork and not for interacting with elders. Depression, anxiety, and other emotional problems can further isolate elders. The most profound separation, however, is the separation from our feelings. In modern Western society, aging, illness, and death are invisible, reflecting our discomfort. For those coping with aging, illness, and death, this invisibility alone can be isolating. Adopting mindfulness practices requires a fundamental shift in attitudes. Mindfulness teaches us to accept painful, pleasurable, and neutral events and feelings with equanimity, knowing they are all temporary.

FREEDOM AND THE FIVE REMEMBRANCES

I am sure to grow old.
I can not avoid aging.
I am sure to become ill.
I can not avoid illness.
I am sure to die.
I can not avoid death.
All things dear and beloved to me.
Are subject to change and separation.

(Thera & Bodhi, 1999, p. 135)

TRY THIS

Find a place to sit quietly and comfortably. Close your eyes and focus on your breath. Spend some time with this practice. Whenever your mind wanders, gently bring your attention back to your breath. After a while, allow the thought of illness and disability to come to you. Perhaps consider the reflection above, a specific situation, or more generally, your feelings about these conditions. Notice not only thoughts as they arise, but physical sensations and emotions. Are there changes in your body? Tightening? Fear? A change in breathing? Allow yourself to sit with these thoughts, feelings, and physical sensations for a while. Notice if they change in intensity, or even come and go. Notice, perhaps, an inclination to push them away or ignore them. If you feel comfortable with it, allow the thought of death to come into your awareness. Your own death or the death of someone you love. Again, notice what arises. Stay with it. Sit with it. Breathe with it. You may try repeating to yourself: "I will grow old; I will face sickness, pain, and death," in any way that feels comfortable and right to you. When you are ready, gradually deepen your breath and come out of the meditation. You may want to end this meditation with a lovingkindness meditation—wishing yourself and others freedom from suffering.

As with all challenging practices, it is important to remember to be kind to ourselves as we stretch our limits. The meditation above, when practiced over time, may increase our comfort level with illness, aging, and death.

Isolated elders may not be able to participate in groups and yet mindfulness can be taught and practiced one to one. It can be as simple, and as challenging, as being *present* in our encounters with our frail elderly clients. Techniques taught in the group format, such as deep breathing, visualization, and simple stretches, can also be taught one to one. More important than the skills taught in the group format is the attitude and presence of the practitioner. This presence can be conveyed in person, via the phone, by CDs and cassettes, and by the Internet. Mindfulness brings increased awareness, compassionate clarity, and informed actions to our work whether in a group setting or in individual work.

ISOLATED ELDERS IN THE NURSING HOME

Overview

Despite living in a congregate setting, many nursing home residents feel isolated. Beyond the reasons stated above, some elders may be confined to their bed for medical reasons and others may have a lifelong history of social isolation. In addition, I have often heard residents say that they did not want to make friends in the nursing home just to lose them. In rural settings, residents may be placed in nursing homes with staff and other residents they have known in the community. In urban settings, it is highly likely that nursing home residents will be placed in an unfamiliar environment among strangers. And the strangers may not even share similar cultures, religions, or backgrounds. Most nursing home residents, however, do participate in groups and relate to each other in the group context. Others may benefit from one-to-one intervention. All of the MBEC practices offered in a group setting can be tailored and individualized.

Susan, Part i

Susan was an 82-year-old widow who had been a nursing home resident for 8 years following an accident that left her with two below-the-knee amputations and killed her husband. She was unable to return to the community and refused to leave her single room. She complained of chronic pain and gradually succumbed to other ailments including congestive heart failure and diabetes mellitus. While physically compromised, Susan was alert and oriented. When I began seeing Susan in her room, I asked her to talk about her pain in some detail.

Elders often feel ignored; listening to their concerns is validating and engages them in the healing process. Health care workers tend to be overworked and rushed. In my individual mindfulness work with residents in the nursing home, I noted two outstanding issues: complaints of pain and the perceived unresponsiveness of staff. Residents felt a lack of control over their situation and dependence on staff, whom they found to be indifferent to their suffering. Mindfulness practice empowers isolated, dependent, and physically suffering clients.

TRY THIS

In conversation with another, listen mindfully. Become aware of your automatic responses and desire to speak, interrupt, or not pay attention. Just as in meditation practice, when we return to the breath over and over and over again, return to the act of listening fully, over and over and over again. If you do respond, do so mindfully, not automatically. Observe even your automatic nonverbal responses to listening. Do you nod? Do you lean forward or back? Check out cues such as arms folded or open. Notice what it is like to listen differently, mindfully.

Allowing residents to articulate and describe their pain, and listening carefully is an intervention in itself. I ask about the location of the pain and the intensity, the duration, and other descriptive factors. I often use an outlined drawing of a figure to enable the resident to specifically indicate areas of pain (Kabat-Zinn, 1990). The resident can choose the color and shape of the pain. I tell residents that they are the experts in their pain; they know what it feels like and what helps. Most can describe what helps—say, an activity, or a conversation with a family. This kind of attention allows me to reflect back to the elder that there were some things in their control that helped. Often, the sense of powerlessness and dependency on medical interventions is so ingrained that elders are not aware of simple things they can do for themselves. This is the mindfulness practice, enabling the patients to listen to their bodies.

SUSAN, PART 2

Susan and I worked together for several sessions in her room. I introduced and demonstrated deep breathing exercises and encouraged her to utilize these when in pain or distress. She had a cassette player that she was able to use, and I gave her a guided meditation tape. Susan was bed bound in the nursing home and expressed her sadness that she could no longer go to the beach. We did a guided imagery, using the beach and her memories of it. Gradually, she reported being able to use these skills on her own and that they were helpful in coping.

Adapted Skills

Guided Imagery

Some nursing home residents are not long-term. Short-term residents come to a nursing home for rehabilitation in hopes that they can return to the community. Groups may be less feasible for this population due to several factors. Rehabilitation therapy and other treatments are the priority, and other appointments often dictate the patient's schedule. Therapy is intensive and tiring, and patients often need to rest when not in therapy. In addition, patients have less incentive to form a group connection since they are focused on discharge. A social work intern described her encounter with a short-term resident: Margaret is a 74-year-old widow on rehabilitation following hip replacement surgery. She is alert and oriented. Staff report she frequently complains of pain.

MARGARET

After leading Margaret in a guided meditation, she remained quiet for a while. I asked her, "How was that for you?" She replied that it was hard to concentrate because of the pain. I asked her if there was any time in which she could focus inward. Her face lit up as she said, "Yes, when you were talking about the ocean waves. I used to love to dive into the ocean waves. I love the ocean. I really should be at the beach. I love sitting on the beach and taking in the sun. I love to watch the sunrise on the beach." I asked her how she felt at the beach. Margaret replied, "Oh I felt powerful and alive. I felt at peace with the fresh air and sunshine. I felt strong." (L. Arnone, personal communication, August 15, 2007)

The guided imagery utilized here is not focused on the present moment, but does allow this short-term resident relief. This imagery also teaches Margaret skills and recalls strengths that she may find useful in healing and restoration.

Meditation and Breath Work

It may help to remind elders who are focused on loss, disability, and pain that their breath is always available to them. Breath awareness meditations can be shortened and simplified, depending on the individual's needs. Elders who are in chronic pain tend to breathe very shallowly. Learning to take a deep breath may be a helpful skill for isolated elders. Others may have respiratory ailments. For these residents, beginning with breath work may not be the best choice. Rather, the meditation focus could be sights, sounds, or other physical sensations (see below).

Body Awareness and Gentle Movement

The body scan and meditation can all be practiced one to one, as appropriate. Elders with multiple medical problems may view their bodies as a foe. The body scan engages us in a more accepting relationship with our bodies as they are. Elders may have an opportunity to consider what works as well as what does not work. Learning a meditation practice may provide moments of peace and also a connection to deeper spiritual roots. Body scans can be abbreviated if the resident is fatigued or medicated. For residents who are missing a limb or have specific areas of pain or intensity, it is helpful not to skip or ignore these issues. For example, if I'm working with a resident who is missing her left leg, I would give her the choice of including the left leg as she remembers it or feels it now. With practice, focusing on their bodies with compassion may allow residents to view their bodies in new ways.

Movement for the Bed Bound

Movements and stretches can be adapted for bed bound elders with a focus on remaining physical abilities. The movements should be very slow, paying attention to the process of moving. I encourage bed bound elders to listen to their bodies and to what feels right for them. Again, I use the basic principles of stretching in all directions and balancing movements. A few suggestions for moving in bed:

- Roll the head from side to side to look at the shoulder.
- Roll shoulders up and back in a circle.
- Curl each finger in and out.
- Extend arms shoulder height and stretch out.
- Lift knees one at a time, extend legs and calves one at a time.
- Practice using a complete breath and regular diaphragmatic breathing. (E. Rosenbaum, personal communication, March 18, 2007)

For further suggestions on yoga stretches for the bed bound, see Appendix A.

Awareness of Senses

Bed bound or isolated nursing home residents may feel that their scope is limited. Mindful awareness can be an excellent tool to open horizons. By paying attention to what is, many doors open. Use what is available and appropriate to encourage the bed bound elder to tune in, mindfully, to their 5 senses. While exploring the senses, it may be useful to also discern the difference

---

TRY THIS: SOUND AWARENESS

Let your eyes close, and rather than focusing on the breath, focus on whatever sounds you hear. There is nothing that you have to do. Let yourself settle back and be receptive to what you hear. Simply hear. If your attention wanders, gently but firmly bring it back to listening. Notice how the sounds arise, change, and fall away. Notice any judgments or thoughts you may have about them. Do this exercise for a few minutes, and when you are ready, open your eyes.

---

between thoughts, feelings, and sensations. They all will arise, but we don't often discriminate. Mindful listening is described above, below mindful tasting and seeing, as well as choiceless awareness are described.

TRY THIS: VISUAL AWARENESS

If you usually meditate with your eyes closed, try keeping your eyes open. Without moving, notice what you see in front of you. Keep your gaze soft, undiscerning. What do you see? What thoughts and feelings arise? Note them and return to your awareness of your vision.

Tasting Awareness

Elders with multiple medical problems may have restrictions on what they may eat or drink. Find out what is possible and work with them. If a resident is on pureed food, try that; if a resident has a restricted diet, use the foods or liquids within the diet. Elana Rosenbaum uses ice chips on the transplant unit with cancer patients (E. Rosenbaum, personal communication, June 3, 2007).

Choiceless Awareness

Opening up to whatever is is a practice. Choiceless awareness is a meditation practice in which the practitioner opens or expands her awareness to include seeing, hearing, and other physical sensations. "You can think of it as simply being receptive to whatever unfolds in each moment" (Kabat-Zinn, 1990, p. 71).

END-OF-LIFE CARE

Witnessing patients at the end of life can present internal and external challenges for caregivers. In the context of a health care model that emphasizes curing, accepting a terminal prognosis can feel like a failure. Our need to fix, or cure, may address our own discomfort with life's realities in the face of a desire to aid another. Mindfulness practice may increase the caregiver's comfort with death and dying and enable the caregiver to be more available to care receivers.

> [T]o enter fully into this place with another asks of us as health professionals a comfort with being in this space with ourselves. Literally a willingness to step into an open, unbounded space one moment after the next, dancing on the edge of chaos while catching the tendency to stray, to revert to old habits, to fill in the empty places. To do something. Anything! Yet helping informed by mindfulness often means *not* doing that which is expected or desired. To do this well, nothing must be promised, save the promise of uncertainty, the open field of possibility. (Santorelli, 1999, p. 139)

The first step is to assess what is needed in each individual situation. Many at the end of life are minimally responsive, focused on the dying process. In these situations it is especially important to attune to nonverbal communication in discerning the appropriate intervention.

ZEN FABLE: A DELICIOUS STRAWBERRY

A monk is taking a walk when he begins to be chased by a hungry tiger. He is fast, but the tiger is faster and is catching up to him. He comes to a cliff and goes over, clutching a vine. The vine, however, is thin and as it stretches, he notices it will soon break, and he will fall to the bottom of a deep ravine. The tiger waits for him on the cliff above. Just then, he notices a plump strawberry growing on the vine. He picks the berry and pops it into his mouth saying, "Ah, delicious!"

The Use of Self

Using words of support, even when there is no response, is generally encouraged. Do not assume the person cannot hear, even though they may not respond. Consider the tone, pacing, and rhythm of your words as well as their content. Tune into the dying person's needs; if they are responsive, ask what helps. The work of dying often takes focus and energy. At times, the most effective intervention is to be present and to offer assistance as needed.

CONSIDER WHEN YOU ARE THINKING ABOUT AN INTERVENTION

Who are you doing this for? Are you focused on the patient's needs or your own? If you find the emotional process too difficult at times, take some time for yourself. Go outside and take a walk. Call a friend. Meditate. Take a bubble bath. Sometimes the best thing we can do for those we care for is to take care of ourselves.

Aromatherapy

Mindfulness creates a supportive environment in which the patient and the caregiver can fully experience sadness, and yet appreciate each available moment. I have also found that using aromatherapy and hand massage benefits both the care receiver and the caregiver. They are relatively easy to learn and to implement. I have often been called to a room by our Palliative Care Team to put in an aromatherapy diffuser. Lavender oil is always my first choice since it is the most researched and accepted essential oil. Families as well as professional caregivers have expressed relief and gratitude for this simple intervention.

Breath Work

In *Coma: The Dreambody Near Death* (1989), Arnold Mindell writes about using the breath as a vehicle for communication with persons at the end of life. Initially the caregiver can observe the rhythm of the patient's breath to determine emotional and physical status. During the end of the dying process, the patient's breath may be erratic; this is normal at this stage. By sitting nearby and perhaps holding the patient's hand, the caregiver can begin to synchronize his or her breath to the patient's. This allows for a connection unavailable otherwise.

Hand Massage

I have found hand massage to be easy to teach and to learn, inexpensive, not time consuming, and widely accepted. Caregivers and care receivers may be more comfortable with hand massage than with a full body massage. In addition, hands are easily accessible, even in bed bound patients. Using a light, rhythmic touch can be relaxing to the caregiver as well as the care receiver. In a recent study, Kolcaba, Dowd, Steiner, & Mitzel (2004) found that while there was no statistically significant effect, the patients receiving the hand massage intervention reported feeling "cared for" and connected to the person providing the massage. Like any informal act, hand massage can be given or received mindfully, just by putting full attention on the massage. A simple stroking hand massage can be easily taught to families who want to communicate their caring nonverbally. Hand massage at the end of life should be very gentle, much more like a stroking than a massage. Nonverbal response to the hand massage should also be monitored to determine any negative response.

Lovingkindness Meditation (Metta)

Connection, mutuality, and presence are at the heart of this practice. Work with what is, focusing on remaining strengths and resources. The lovingkindness meditation, as described in Chapter 2, may be a good procedure with end-of-life patients. You can say it out loud with them, if they are open to it, or you may say it to yourself, wishing them to be happy and free from suffering. These phrases should be adapted and modified when needed; the deeper intention is to connect with our compassionate self.

HOMEBOUND ELDERS

A Telephone Mindfulness Group

The plagues of loneliness, helplessness, and boredom may also visit homebound elders. Elders often prefer to stay at home despite their disabilities. At times, however, it means the elder is isolated in his or her home, perhaps with a professional caregiver who may share no common heritage. Rural elders are more frequently at risk. Technology may provide a means to communicate through distance learning. Many elders are becoming increasingly comfortable with technology; future generations will be even more comfortable. While not targeting elders specifically, Steve Flowers (n.d.) runs an online MBSR class with implications for this population.

Consider a telephone support group as a way of working with elders and other homebound individuals. Conference calls can be set up through phone companies, and group members will need to be available at the selected time. I have offered a 5-week, 50-minute class for six-to-eight homebound participants. I premailed audio practice cassettes, selected readings, and drawings to illustrate deep breathing and yoga poses. On the phone, I gave instructions on the mindfulness practices and then asked group members to try them. For the yoga poses, group members would listen to the instructions, and then put down the phone and practice the pose. Following this, group members returned to the phone and asked questions or shared feedback. These classes included weekly homework assignments of practicing what we learned. In this class, I included deep breathing, mindfulness, visualization, modified yoga, and lovingkindness meditation.

Group members were increasingly interactive as the class progressed. Group members also verbalized benefits from the exercises even though they were not physically in the same room. Allowing for a quiet meditation while on the phone was initially disconcerting, but ultimately satisfying. I had assumed that the visual cues and the physical presence of the group members in the more traditional groups and settings provided teaching information and a sense of connection. Yet, a sense of connection developed in this telephone group also, even though members were physically separated, as far as New York City and Florida.

At the group's conclusion, class members reported continued use of the skills, especially the deep breathing. Most also expressed an interest in ongoing similar groups. One participant, Ms. C, stated that during the past 6 years, the mindfulness "guidance and your wonderful tape kept me alive and helped me to become the real person I am today. Without your help I never would have reached my 90th birthday, and had the courage to go to Florida after my dear son passed."

Tapes and CDs

Tapes and CDs are another excellent medium for sharing mindfulness practices with frail elders. Homebound elders in a long-term home health care program are offered tapes by visiting social workers. The social worker introduces the tape and sits with the elder and the caregiver for the initial experience. The tapes are left with them, providing an opportunity for a shared experience, benefiting both caregiver and care receiver. In addition, for those working with a culturally diverse population, guided tapes have been translated.

I also have tapes available for agitated residents on a dementia unit. The tapes are tailored for this population and use my familiar voice. The language is simple, concrete, repetitive, and slow, with a focus on tone, pacing, and affect. While not all persons with dementia have responded well to the use of headsets, one agitated resident was captivated by the tapes. Staff found that this resident was able to focus and respond to the guided meditations on the CD. Resources for mindfulness CDs, as well as guided meditations that can be the basis for making your own, are listed Appendix B and F.

CONCLUSION

The suffering of isolated elders is compounded by their isolation. Kabat-Zinn describes his adaptations of MBSR in this way: "The challenge we are faced with . . . is how to make use of a vocabulary, structure and format that will invite people into the deep practice of meditation. . . . Meditation is not a collection of techniques that belongs to any group. It is a way of being" (Kabat-Zinn, 2005, p. 33). In the same way, for elders and their caregivers, these practices, if presented in a way that is accessible, may offer a way of being that mitigates their suffering.

REFERENCES

Flowers, S. (n.d.) *Mindfulness-Based Stress Reduction online class offerings.* Retrieved July 30, 2007, from http://www.mindfullivingprograms.com/onlinecourse.php

Kabat-Zinn, J. (1990). *Full catastrophe living: Using the wisdom of your body and mind to face stress, pain and illness.* New York: Dell.

Kabat-Zinn, J. (2005, May). In B. Boyce (author). The man who prescribes the medicine of the moment. *Shambhala Sun,* pp. 29–35.

Kolcaba, K., Dowd, T., Steiner, R., & Mitzel, A. (2004). Efficacy of hand massage for enhancing the comfort of hospice patients. *Journal of Hospice and Palliative Nursing,* 6(2), 91–101.

Mindell, A. (1989). *Coma: The dreambody near death.* London: Penguin.

Santorelli, S. (1999). *Heal thy self.* New York: Bell Tower.

Thera, N., & Bodhi, B. (Trans. & Eds.). (1999). *Numerical discourses of the Buddha: An anthology of Suttas from the Anguttara Nikaya.* Walnut Creek, CA: AltaMira.

Thomas, W. H. (2004). *What are old people for? How elders will save the world.* Acton, MA: VanderWyk & Burnham.

CHAPTER 8

Dance Like Nobody Is Watching: Mindfulness-Based Elder Care and Creativity

Dance like nobody's watching; love like you've never been hurt. Sing like nobody's listening; live like it's heaven on earth.

—Mark Twain

Creativity serves us in many ways. Creativity can connect where words no longer make sense. Creativity can help all of us make sense of our world, allowing deeper understanding and healing. During the process of creation, that which is deep within us finds voice, expressing itself through art, poetry, music, movement, and other creative activities. The creative experience is often mindful. As we concentrate on creating, our mind, body, and spirit unite. In addition, witnessed creativity may be equally engaging. We can be fully present while reading, listening to music, observing art, drama, or dance. Our sense of time may change. We may feel a new openness and curiosity about the world. We may experience a new perspective on our world and experience new insights. Creative groups can also generate community. Through the creative process, we learn new things about ourselves and find meaning where we may have been uncertain. We all are creative beings, and yet many of us feel we are not, cutting off this resource within ourselves. Creativity is not limited by cognition; in fact, cognition may inhibit creativity as we screen out "mistakes."

This chapter specifically describes creative interventions utilized with elders. Creativity is explored in the context of the senses (hearing, sight, touch, taste, and smell), movement, and mindfulness practice. These exercises can provide an avenue for reminiscence for elders with limited cognition of their roots and memories. Elders with profound memory loss bring back words to a

---

THINK ABOUT THIS

How many of us would have learned to walk if we had the same fears of making mistakes or seeming foolish as we do now? When you begin a new creative project, imagine yourself as a child and allow yourself to fall down, get up, and fall down again. Care about the process, not the product of creating. Learn to laugh at yourself.

---

song from their youth. The smell of bread baking or flowers from a childhood home may trigger memories. The creative use of our senses can remind those with frailties of that which is still available to them. It can also open avenues of communication and expression. While mindfulness precepts encourage practitioners to stay in the present moment, reminiscence encourages elders to reconnect with their past, informing who they are in the present.

Talented social work interns under my supervision and other creative therapists developed the interventions described below. They may be used as models, if appropriate. Or, consider your population and what inspires you.

VISUAL ARTS

Feelings Art Group

In 2000, two social work interns under my supervision initiated a group for residents on the dementia unit to incorporate art as a way of expressing and sharing feelings. The group size ranged from 4–9 members, and the membership was fairly consistent. Group participants were asked to identify on a "Mood Thermometer" whether they felt happy, neutral, or sad. The Mood Thermometer had three simple faces with expressions to reflect these three moods. Residents could say how they felt or point to a face. This exercise was designed to verbally and nonverbally engage these confused residents and encourage identification and expression of their feelings, not to evaluate outcomes.

The primary modality of the group was visual arts, and group leaders focused on how the residents were feeling in the present moment. Conceptualized as single sessions, the group offered an art activity, often accompanied by another sensory stimulus such as music, aromatherapy, or touch. The leaders encouraged discussion on the group's theme of the day. Themes included seasons, "who I love," "what I believe," marriage, the sea, "how music makes me feel," and "what I like to eat." Group leaders reported that this group helped members to find a voice for their feelings. Members exhibited increased ability to verbalize feelings during the group and increased their interactions among group members. The following quotes from group members demonstrate the impact of the interventions on these elders with dementia:

Group Connections

Ms. N. turned to Ms. R and said, "I know you are one of us." Ms. R responded, "I wouldn't be anything else" (Bober, McClellan, McBee, & Westreich, 2002, p. 82).

Reminiscence

In response to the activity "What I believe," Ms. V said, "My mother has twelve children. When she died, they put her in the ground, but I don't know where my mother was. Up to this day, I don't know where my mother is. I'd have to dig, dig, dig." "You miss her," the group facilitator responded. "I shake," Ms. V replied (Bober et al., 2002, pp. 82–83).

Expression of Strong Feelings

During Valentine's Day, the group focused on "Who I love."

Ms. S said, "I love Mary." She repeated this many times even singing about her love for her sister Mary. With a crayon, she traced a heart and struggled to write "Mary" on the page below. "I love them all," she said. "Mary is my little sister . . . Mary! Oh Mary! I love my little Mary!" These creative exercises clearly allowed the often-confused group members to reminisce about important life experiences and important human connections (Bober et al., 2002, p. 83).

Communication Through Pictures

Art or visual memories can also be passively stimulated. The story below illustrates the use of a photo to evoke a memory in a profoundly demented elder.

Visual Memories

A very confused and verbally agitated resident was working with a social work intern. He researched her birthplace on the Internet and found a photo of a bridge in the area of Germany where she grew up. When viewing the photo, the resident became animated and clearly articulated that she used to walk on that bridge with her father.

POETRY AND WORDS

A social work intern began a group for frail elders using words to stimulate memory and conversation. She wrote single words and simple phrases in large, bold print on cardboard, which she covered with clear contact paper. The group of nursing home residents gathered around a table and selected words. The initial conception was that the group would write poetry with the words. This activity was to allow group members to express and share emotions that they might not have been willing to articulate explicitly. The intern had noticed that more traditional talk groups sometimes privileged the outspoken and became stale in repetition. Offering this tactile and creative activity did not require sophisticated language skills and created space and support for less verbal individuals to get involved. The participants, a group of residents with physical and cognitive frailties, did not create poetry, but did find the words a helpful starting point for the expression of powerful feelings.

POETRY IN THE NURSING HOME

One group member, usually quiet and confused, "had in front of her words that evoked springtime—maybe grass, sunshine, or joy. Without prompting, she began to share a story about living on a farm in England during the Second World War. Apparently, she met and had a romantic relationship with a soldier in the springtime, near her home on a farm. The memory was highly detailed, and, in a normally somber group, quite titillating. Her entire mood changed as she was transported back in time to this wonderful memory from her youth. "I recall having visions of cows in pasture, the smell of freshly cut grass, the romantic tension between two young people." Another man "was notoriously cranky and sneered at my efforts to draw him in. So I left him alone, and from the corner of my eye, I watched him arranging and rearranging the words in front of him. And I noticed that he listened intently to what the others said" (S. Segal-McCaslin, personal communication, August 8, 2007).

MUSIC

Elders can both listen to and participate in music. I have used classical or calming music during some groups to create a healing milieu. Meditators may use ritual to set their intention for practice. For some, the use of incense, altars, photos of teachers, or other sacred paraphernalia may establish a stronger connection to practice. Mindfulness practice is about accepting what is. The institutional environment is a fixed part of life for residents. Leaving the environment is rarely an option. For institutionalized elders, subtly changing the environment with music and aromatherapy is possible and may trigger memories of the group and meditative experience that allows for positive memories and reinforcement.

In a group for elders with dementia, I use classical or other calming music to ease the agitation that often exists on these floors. Breathing exercises and gentle movement can be done to this music. At other times, I use salsa and music from the Caribbean to inspire more energized movement and participation. Group members are given tambourines and rattles to shake and are encouraged to move in or out of their chairs. Residents who rarely respond to other interventions will shake a rattle, move a little, or smile at others dancing. This exercise usually engages staff also, and they will come in and dance with the residents.

I have found music to be a language in which communication is possible when other forms of communication are not. At times, I mirror the elders' rhythm, at others I do a call and answer. In a group setting, elders may feel connected to each other through the music. Music can also lead to natural movement as we experience it in our bodies. This activity can be helpful for those having difficulty with balance, gait, fluid movement, range of motion, and fine and gross motor skills. Singing lyrics may aid those with speech difficulties. Music can affect mood, aiding those with anxiety, pain, and depression.

Music also triggers memories. Identify culturally appropriate music for your elders and groups. Elders with advanced dementia have been known to remember the words to childhood songs (Tomaino, 1999, 2000).

> I learned so much from M . . . , really almost every day. I learned that before the music started she had no idea where she was. She was unfailingly polite and said nice things about her surroundings but never really knew where she was. But when I started a song, she was in by the 3rd or 4th note, and THAT's when she knew where she was. Every word, every note, confident, happy, safe, totally herself. She was a gift to me for the insight she gave me about the power of music. (J. Hitchcock, personal communication, September 13, 2007)

Humming and singing to music can offer benefits beyond reminiscence. The vibrations that happen when we sing exercise our internal organs and may increase the balance and harmony in our lives. The yoga of sound, a less well-known aspect of yoga, identifies the unique benefits of different sounds within us (Paul, 2004).

MOVEMENT AND MUSIC

TRY THIS

Find a private space and close the door so you will not be interrupted. Put on music that you love and start moving. Let the movements initiate internally without preconception. Just move. Nobody is watching, so don't think about how you look, just move in any way you feel. Have fun, express your feelings in movement. Move slowly or quickly, move your entire body, just let the music move you from the inside out. After a few minutes, stop and stand still. Quietly notice how you are feeling.

Movement and music naturally go together. I have found that this is the area in which I can be most playful. As group leader, if I allow myself to be silly and laugh at myself, the group loses its inhibitions also. Elders can be great teachers here. Kinesthetic movements can reconnect us with nonverbal memories. As mentioned in Chapter 6, elders with memory loss respond well to both mirroring my movements and to movements that trigger memories:

Imitating Body Movements as Exercise

Rocking a baby: strengthens the arms and rotates the shoulders.
Playing the piano: exercises all the fingers. The tapping on the table can also be a tai chi release of energy.
Shaking water off the hands and arms: loosens up the body parts shaken, gets us silly.
Washing hair: scalp massage.
Swimming: arm and shoulder movements.
Walking: leg movements in a chair.
Other fun movements:
Open and close like flowers: breathing in and opening the arms wide, breathing out and hugging ourselves. When we hug ourselves we can also give our shoulders a little massage.
Breathing in and using our arms in a gathering motion to bring in what we want, naming it—love, energy, healing. Breathing out and pushing away what we don't want: pain, sadness.

I often encourage the use of sounds with all this activity. Consider varying the movement, timing, pace, intensity, rhythm, as well as engaging all the body parts, moving in various ways, and in different directions (up, down, sideways). Again, the most important intervention is you, the leader. Mindfulness is not only practiced in stillness, but also in motion. It is important to be open and in touch with your own inner movement. It is not important to be graceful, perfect, or a trained dancer. In fact, your imperfections and sense of humor can inspire the group to lose their inhibitions. And their joy may inspire you!

TOUCH

Touch is an important sensation for elders. Elders, especially institutionalized elders, are frequently touched while personal care is provided. Care providers, however, are often rushed and impatient. In past practice, nurses offered back rubs. This custom is rarely provided now. I offer gentle hand massages, shoulder rubs, and hugs regularly. As with all interventions, it is important to be sensitive to each individual's verbal and nonverbal response to physical closeness; nevertheless, I have rarely found an elder who does not respond positively to touch. Appendix C details a gentle hand massage that I have successfully used and taught. I also may incorporate self-massage into group movement exercises.

The sensation of touch can encompass the use of the senses mindfully. Consider bringing objects with different tactile qualities to residents. Fabrics can provide a large range of textures including rough, silky, and velvety. I have used objects from nature such as flowers, shells, or leaves.

TASTE AND SMELL

The use of objects to stimulate taste and smell may also kindle memories or awareness of the present moment. The smell of food can trigger memories or appetite. In some nursing homes, a bread maker is used for this purpose. Many elders lose some of their taste awareness, but may respond to the stronger smells of fresh garlic or lemons. The response may be nonverbal, but the memory will be aroused nonetheless.

FLOWERS

Ms. B., a nursing home resident on the dementia unit, was rarely verbal. During one session of the Feelings Art Group, facilitators brought flowers and gave them out to group members to experience.

They were encouraged to smell, touch, and see the flowers. Ms. B was given a rose, which she smelled. "The flower triggered an immediate emotional response: her eyes filled with tears and she began to weep. Ms. B. was able to communicate to the group, with help from the co-leaders, that the scent of the rose reminded her of a place from her past that was no longer there" (Bober et al., p. 84).

USE OF NATURE

The best things in life are nearest. Breath in your nostrils, light in your eyes, flowers at your feet, duties at your hand, the path of right just before you.
                                                    —Robert Louis Stevenson

Elders, especially institutionalized elders, are often removed from nature. Nature can be a wonderful resource for healing and renewal, and yet physical and environmental obstacles may prevent access to this resource. Nursing homes weigh the risk/benefit of elopement and safety and may restrict the elders' movements to protect themselves and the elders. As Culture Change impacts these environments and regulators accept the Pioneer Network credo that "Life involves risk," this attitude may change. For the meantime, consider bringing nature inside for those who can no longer get outside. In *Bring Me the Ocean: Nature as Teacher, Messenger, and Intermediary,* Reynolds shares her experiences bringing nature into hospitals, prisons, and libraries. She finds that nature can restore and heal, providing a sense of mystery and well-being.

> At a chronic care hospital we met Irene, an elderly, Greek woman. Able to speak only her native Greek, she had become isolated by her inability to communicate with other residents. Over recent years she had gradually lapsed into silence. . . .
> On this day we came with an ocean program. Along with sand and shells, we brought thick piles of seaweed indoors. When Irene saw the seaweed being lifted up out of the buckets, she wheeled her chair over, her expression shifting profoundly.
> Picking up handfuls of kelp, Irene smelled its saltiness and began weeping. Slowly, haltingly, she began to speak. Some of us understood her Greek, but we all understood her. Such beauty lit her face as she poured forth descriptions of the ocean and her childhood home! (Reynolds, 1995, p. xi)

As an adjunct to guided imagery, I bring in seashells and beach rocks for residents to hold while I play a CD of wave sounds. I may ask them to visualize the beach with these aids, describing the beach smells, sounds, sights, and physical sensations.

TOYS

Using toys can assist in communicating mindfulness skills and also help to remind us to be playful. Some toys I have used are:

Pinwheels: residents can practice breathing a long, slow exhale while attempting to get the pinwheel to spin.

Bubbles: they also remind elders to breathe slowly and steadily. And, they can be fun to watch! Elders may try to grab them, stretching as they reach.

Balloons: they are fun for batting around. They can provide exercise, range of motion stretches, and eye–hand coordination.

Elastics: looping together a series of elastics can provide an exercise aid that stretches with some resistance.

All of the toys may also lead to our last intervention: laughter and humor!

HUMOR

Jean Vanier, the founder of l'Arche, communities of those with mental disabilities and those who share a life with them, views disabilities as universal and acknowledgment of disabilities as strength. In his acceptance speech for the Dignitas Humana Award on October 25, 2000, Jean Vanier describes an encounter with a "normal." He states that normals are known for having problems with work, family, and life. Mr. Normal is discussing his problems with Jean Vanier when Jean Claude, one of the Down syndrome residents, burst into the room, laughing. He shook the hands of both Jean Vanier and his visitor and left the room still laughing.

> And Mr. Normal turned to me and he said, "Isn't it sad, children like that."
> He couldn't see that Jean Claude was a happy guy. It's a blindness, and it's an inner blindness which is the most difficult to heal. (Vanier, 2000)

Humor and laughter may seem to be the easiest intervention, but for many of us "normals," it may be the hardest. Like everything, we can improve with practice. Why not start with a smile?

Once you have begun smiling more, try laughing. You may need aids like jokes or funny movies at the beginning. One way to initiate laughter in groups is just to start. Or a group member may begin laughing in a way that is contagious to you or others. Keep it up for a few minutes, building to a crescendo and slowly coming down. When the room becomes quiet, just sit with the

---

TRY THIS

Smile; notice what happens. Keep doing it throughout the day. Notice if your mood or thoughts change when you do it.

---

quiet for a while and see how it feels. Another option is to ask participants to put their hands on their bellies and laugh. They can begin by just saying, "Ha, ha, ha" or "Ho, ho, ho." You can also go around the group and ask different members to laugh and then ask the group to imitate this unique laughter (L. Sierra, personal communication, August 10, 2007). It is okay if it feels forced at first. Sometimes, this activity becomes mirthful, and genuine laughter breaks out. For me, laughter is a genuinely connecting experience. We are not teacher and taught, helper and helped; we are just two—or more—people laughing together. When working with elders, remember the opportunity *you* have to be healed through laughter and by heartfelt connection.

REFERENCES

Bober, S., McClellan, E., McBee, L., & Westreich, L. (2002). The Feelings Art Group: A vehicle for personal expression in skilled nursing home residents with dementia. *Journal of Social Work in Long-Term Care, 1*(4), 73–87.

Paul, R. (2004). *The yoga of sound: Healing and enlightenment through the sacred practice of mantra.* Novato, CA: New World Library.

Reynolds, R. A. (1995). *Bring me the ocean: Nature as teacher, messenger, and intermediary.* Acton, MA: VanderWyk & Burnham.

Tomaino, C. M. (1999). Active music therapy approaches for neurologically impaired patients. In C. D. Maranto (Ed.), *Music therapy and medicine: Theoretical and clinical applications* (pp. 115–122). American Music Therapy Association.

Tomaino, C. M. (2000). Working with images and recollection with elderly patients. In D. Aldridge (Ed.), *Music Therapy in Dementia* (pp. 195–211). London: Jessica Kingsley.

Twain, M. (n.d.). Retrieved August 12, 2007, from http://www.quotedb.com/quotes/2338

Vanier, J. (2000, October 25). *Signs of hope for the new millennium.* Acceptance Speech for the Dignitas Humana Award presented at St. John's University. Retrieved August 5, 2007, from http://speakingoffaith.publicradio.org/programs/larche/particulars.shtml

SECTION III

Caregivers

CHAPTER 9

Who Will Take Care of Us? An Overview of Mindfulness-Based Elder Care for Caregivers

- "'Caregiver syndrome' [is] a new term to describe the symptoms of stress for full-time caregivers." (LeRoy, 2007)
- Elderly caregivers are at a 63 percent higher risk of mortality than non-caregivers in the same age group. (Schulz & Beach, 1999)
- "Most [nursing assistants in long-term care] workers are relatively disadvantaged economically and have low levels of educational attainment. While these paraprofessional workers are engaged in physically and emotionally demanding work, they are among the lowest paid in the service industry, making little more than the minimum wage." (Stone & Wiener, 2001)
- Increasingly, policymakers, providers, consumers and researchers describe the attempts to employ and retain nursing assistants to care for frail elders as a "crisis." (Stone, 2001)

The growth in the aging population has implications for both formal and informal caregiving. An increased population with chronic illness and disability will require more caregivers. Informal caregivers provide care for family members and friends without pay. Formal or professional caregivers are paid employees or volunteers connected with a service provider. There are differences between these groups, but one important commonality is that those who provide the direct care for elders have the most impact on elders' lives. Another commonality is that caregiving is stressful. Caregiving for persons with dementia and behavioral problems is recognized to be the most stressful (Pinquart & Sörensen, 2003).

The emotional and physical impact of caregiving is well documented (Cohen-Mansfield, 1995; Schulz & Martire, 2004; Vitaliano, Zhang, & Scanlan, 2003). The well-being of care receivers and caregivers is also linked in many ways. The moods and conditions of caregivers and care receivers closely impact each other. Care provision is usually an intimate experience; frail elders are often dependent on others for personal needs and for their very survival. For caregivers, the tasks can be physically and emotionally taxing. Financial constraints are often part of this picture: informal caregivers are unpaid and may have other responsibilities including paid employment. Direct care professional caregivers for elders are poorly paid, tend to be less satisfied with their jobs, and to have secondary health problems. These conditions often lead to increased job turnover, sick days, and poor job performance (Dunn, Rout, Carson, & Ritter, 1994; Pekkarinen, Sinervo, Perälä, & Elovainio, 1990; Zimmerman et al., 2005). Despite similar interests, there are also differences between paid and unpaid caregivers, and research studies focus on these populations separately. This section discusses mindfulness groups and other interventions for both formal and informal caregivers. This chapter provides a brief overview of the impact of caregiving on informal and formal caregivers as well as interventions proven to be helpful.

INFORMAL CAREGIVERS

Who Are Informal Caregivers?

Family and friends are often the first line of defense in caregiving. It can be as simple as checking in by phone or as consuming as 24-hour supervision and personal care. Informal caregiving has changed as our health, life expectancy, and lifestyles have changed. Large families living in close proximity or in the same house are rare. In addition, most adults work long hours outside the home. Elders who live into their 90s may need care from their children who are in their 60s or 70s and who may have their own health problems.

Informal caregivers can be any age, ethnicity, or gender. Women, especially daughters, are more likely to be caregivers. Informal caregivers are relied on heavily not only by their families, but also by government agencies that would have to shoulder the burden in their absence. Programs supporting informal caregivers are inadequate as is recognition of their services and sacrifices (Feinberg & Newman, 2006; Wolff & Kasper, 2006). Currently, it is estimated that from 5.9 to 52 million caregivers in the United States assist family and friends with everyday activities. These figures vary based on the definition of *caregiver* and *care receiver*, including the age of the care receiver, the number of hours of care provided, the type of care, and the length of time care is provided (Family Caregiver Alliance, 2001).

How Does Caregiving Impact the Informal Caregivers' Lives?

In a recent article, Wolff and Kasper (2006) noted that 52.8% of caregivers provide assistance by themselves, without support from a secondary caregiver. In addition, 41.3% are children of the care receiver, and most likely employed full time; 38.4% are spouses who may also be elders with their own frailties. Individual personalities and situations differ, but studies report that informal caregivers experience more depression and other mental health problems than their noncaregiving peers (Covinsky et al., 2003; Schulz, O'Brien, Bookwals, & Fleissner, 1995). Nursing home placement of the care receiver may actually worsen depression and anxiety disorders for the caregiver. Spouse caregivers find this transition the most difficult, and almost half continue to visit the care receiver daily (Schulz et al., 2004).

Common Themes for Informal Caregivers of Frail Elders

Isolation

The intensity of the tasks of caregiving combined with other responsibilities held by the caregiver may isolate them from the very support that could mitigate the impact of caregiving. Caregivers may also feel emotionally isolated if there is no one who understands their feelings.

Anger

Anger can be an underlying theme, since it is unsanctioned by society and made more toxic because the caregiver may not be able to share this emotion. It may lead to further isolation and, potentially, to health problems (Vitaliano, Scanlan, Krenz, & Fujtmoto, 1996). Anger may be realistically focused on the unfair burdens of caregiving when families do not respond equally to the tasks. Anger at the care receiver for demanding, nonsensical, and dangerous behaviors can also become anger at oneself for not being more compassionate or understanding (Tabak, Ehrenfeld, & Alpert, 1997).

Despair, Uncertainty, and Fear

Caring for elders with chronic conditions does not usually bode well, as the elder will usually not get better and generally will become more disabled and require more care. Care needs may change daily, rapidly, or slowly. The children of frail elders, who may be elders themselves, may wonder what does this mean for me? Will I get this disease?

Perception of Stress

The caregiver's stress level is more likely to be associated with his or her perception of the tasks than the type and extent of caregiving. Yates, Tennstedt, and Chang (1999) found that for informal caregivers of elders, a higher level of a "sense of mastery" lowered the risk of depression. Goodman, Zarit, and Steiner (1997) found that the caregiver's evaluation of the caregiving experience was a factor in caregiver strain.

Physical Demands

Caregiving for elders may also be physically demanding. Elders may need help with transferring from chair to bed, or they may need assistance getting onto the toilet, for example. If the elder is confused, he or she may be combative, striking out at the caregiver. These tasks may also lead to injury for caregivers.

Caregiving Rewards

Caregivers also report important rewards from the caregiving experience, including feeling appreciated and helpful. Some even find their relationship with the care receiver improved (Beach, Schulz, Yee, & Jackson, 2000).

What Helps? Support for Informal Caregivers

A review of the literature on interventions for informal caregivers of elders with dementia by Schultz and colleagues found that small to moderate effects have been reported in many studies. While few studies report clinically significant outcomes, the interventions still hold promise for mitigating the profound and pervasive health and psychological impacts of caregiving (Schulz et al., 2002). A review of caregiver research by Mittleman (2005) found that psychoeducational interventions were the most utilized, while supportive interventions were more effective in relieving psychological symptoms for both caregivers and care receivers. In sum, she found that treating caregivers was an important aspect of the overall therapy for chronic diseases and disabilities.

Counseling and support groups alone have been found to be effective in diminishing depression in spouse-caregivers of Alzheimer's disease patients.

The alleviation was sustained for over 3 years following the groups and one-to-one support (Mittelman, Roth, Coon, & Haley, 2004). Mutual care support groups allow persons with similar life challenges to connect in a safe and supported environment. Caregivers come to groups for respite, socialization, ventilation, validation, education, skills, and hope (Toseland, 1995, p. 228). They may, however, neglect their own care needs for many reasons. They may feel that they need to be vigilant, worrying that if they do not constantly monitor the care receiver's condition there will be disastrous consequences. They may also feel guilty about enjoying pleasures denied to the care receiver. It may be difficult to make plans if the care receiver's condition is unstable. Caregivers may need encouragement and skills to care for themselves. Just committing to a group can take courage and initiative.

FORMAL CAREGIVERS

Professionals who care for elders are also a mixed group. Direct care workers, who provide the brunt of the care, tend to be lower in socioeconomic class and education and are overwhelmingly female. The pay is poor, and the physical and emotional demands are high (Personick, 1990; Stone & Wiener, 2001). Job turnover for nursing assistants in long-term care is estimated at 40–100% annually (Cohen-Mansfield, 1997; Stone & Wiener, 2001). Turnover adds increased job stress to those who stay, and the cycle may continue. Federal and state regulations dictate most of the job responsibilities and are perceived, often correctly, as paper compliance. This situation increases the frustration of caregivers who are often prevented from spending time with elders in order to complete paperwork. The position of direct caregiver allows them to understand the unique needs of each resident. Relationships often develop when care is provided over a number of years. And yet, these caregivers are traditionally not engaged in decision making and may even be penalized for not following procedure. They also may provide care for persons of different races or backgrounds from themselves, leading to cultural misunderstandings. Studies on stress and professional caregivers cite time pressure (Pekkarinen, Sinervo, Perälä, & Elovainio, 2004), poor wages, understaffing, feeling unvalued by management, physically demanding work (Dunn et al., 1994), high resident demand, management policies, and personal problems (Cohen-Mansfield, 1995). Unfortunately, there is less research on effective interventions for formal caregivers. In fact, the term *caregiver* is usually assumed to mean informal caregivers.

Culture Change initiatives value and seek actively to engage direct care workers. Focusing on a person-centered, creative, and individualized model of care, proponents of Culture Change view relationships as central to care provision. (See "Pioneer Values" in Chapter 1.) The Paraprofessional Healthcare

Institute focuses both on the caregiver and the care receiver, acknowledging the intrinsic link between the two. Bill Thomas, founder of the Eden Alternative, defines the first step in changing the way nursing homes care for frail elders is to "treat the staff the way they want the staff to treat the elders" (Thomas, 2002). Research on the problems of recruitment and retention and the reasons cited for these problems also point to solutions. Interventions that offer stress reduction and also empower caregivers may begin to effect a change.

MINDFULNESS GROUPS FOR FORMAL AND INFORMAL CAREGIVERS

To date, there are no published studies determining the effectiveness of mindfulness training for informal or formal caregivers of frail elders. In 2006, Minor, Carlson, Mackenzie, and Zernicke reported results from an 8-week MBSR course for 44 informal caregivers of young children with chronic conditions. Following the course, caregivers experienced significant decreases in stress symptoms and mood disturbance. Informal practices that could be used and integrated into busy demanding schedules were reported to be particularly helpful. Members also reported benefiting from the skills and health promotional aspects of this course. Half-day sessions were discontinued, however, due to poor attendance. No control group was offered for this study.

In Sweden, a pilot study documented the responses of 52 health care professionals who participated in a 50-hour program in mindfulness exercises, cognitive attitude training, and lectures (Schenström, Rönnberg, & Bodlund, 2006). Homework and formal and informal exercises were all included in this program, which focused on teaching caregivers to care for themselves through mindfulness practice. Levels of mindfulness, perceived quality of life, and well-being increased during the program and persisted at 3 months. Within the experimental group, perception of stress in and outside the workplace decreased.

Stress Reduction Classes for Caregivers

Research has also documented positive effects of other models of stress reduction for caregivers of frail elders. One study reports on classes with modifications to the format to allow for the time constraints of these caregivers, and with more targeted discussions on caregiving for elders (López, Crespo, & Zarit, 2007). The caregivers in two experimental groups participated in a stress management program as an 8-week, individual, traditional intervention or in a minimal-therapist-contact (MTC) format. The MTC format provides skill training and support via phone, brief meetings, manuals, and audiovisual material. A control group was wait-listed. Participants in the traditional program experienced higher reductions in anxiety and depression than did the MTC and wait-listed control groups. The MTC group also benefited, although to a lesser extent.

In a pilot study published in 2004, Waelde, Thompson, and Gallagher-Thompson describe a six-session yoga and (mantra-focused) meditation class offered to 12 Caucasian and Latina informal caregivers for elders with dementia. Although there was no control group, depression and anxiety were significantly reduced and mastery was significantly improved in participants. Burns, Nichols, Martindale-Adams, Graney, and Lummus (2003) developed and studied two, 2-year interventions with informal caregivers of those with Alzheimer's disease. One group of caregivers was given educational materials on behavior management; the other group received these materials plus caregiver stress-coping. The caregivers who received the behavior management without the stress coping information were found to have significantly worse outcomes for general well-being and a trend toward increased risk of depression.

Although studies on interventions for staff are less common, D'Eramo, Papp, and Rose (2001) reported on a group in which nursing assistants in long-term care were taught meditation, yoga, cognitive techniques, healing touch, and spirituality. Participants in this small sample reported that they planned to use the skills personally and with their patients and families. These researchers also report that administrative buy-in is an essential component of this training.

Benefits for Caregiver and Care Recipient

Interventions that benefit caregivers will also benefit the care recipient. A study targeting caregivers for other populations demonstrates the effectiveness of mindfulness training for both caregivers and care receivers. Singh et al. (2004) measured happiness in care receivers with multiple disabilities when cared for by caregivers with and without mindfulness training. Care receivers happiness evidenced marked increases when cared for by individuals who participated in an 8-week mindfulness program.

There is also substantial documentation of the opposite: caregivers who are stressed, depressed, and angry provide poor, and sometimes, abusive, care. One study found that potentially harmful behavior was more likely from spouses or when the care receiver was cognitively impaired or had great care needs. Documented behaviors included "screaming and yelling, insulting or swearing, threatening to send to a nursing home, and withholding food" (Beach et al., 2005, p. 255).

MINDFULNESS-BASED ELDER CARE

Mindfulness-Based Elder Care courses were initially offered to nursing home residents. Over time, I noticed that staff would often sit nearby and observe, sometimes even practice the skills along with the residents. Eventually, some staff asked to sit in on the sessions. It made sense that by teaching caregivers to manage their own stress, they might be more patient and less stressed with their care receivers. In the beginning, we offered a 1-hour program to all interdisciplinary staff in the nursing home. The program introduced the mind-body connection, simple, deep breathing, and relaxation exercises. The response was positive. Subsequently, a 7-week MBEC course was offered to approximately 100 staff members. Again, qualitative reports were overwhelmingly positive. Staff retention on the units that participated in the class was 100%, and nursing staff satisfaction showed improvement.

Mindfulness groups offered to informal family and friend caregivers can also provide skills and support. Informal caregivers frequently report stress and stress-related illness. Mindfulness groups encourage self-care in the context of care provision. In an informal caregiver MBEC group, many participants reported a decrease in somatic complaints and an increase in satisfaction in the caregiving role. Caregivers could be "in the moment" with their loved one, rather than worrying about the past or future.

Kabat-Zinn recommends that MBSR program participants be a medically heterogeneous population. He suggests that this configuration better enables participants to understand the larger commonalities of the human condition (Kabat-Zinn, 1996). I have held both homogeneous and heterogeneous caregiver groups, and found that both had benefits. While my caregiver groups were not specifically for participants with medical problems, they were specifically for either formal or informal caregivers. Caregiver groups build on understood commonalities. Adaptations made for these groups also target mutual time restraints. The caregiving process is significant for its consumption of time, and caregivers, both formal and informal, consistently report a lack of spare time. I also hold programs that are open to residents, formal and informal caregivers, and paid private companions. These programs are noteworthy in that participants represent extremely diverse levels of cognition and physical frailty. In this context, practicing meditation, yoga, and mindfulness together focuses on the commonalities remaining rather than on disabilities. This section details these programs.

CONSIDER THIS

Every 72 seconds someone in America develops Alzheimer's (Alzheimer's Association, n.d.).

REFERENCES

Alzheimer's Association. (n.d.). *Alzheimer's disease facts and figures. A statistical abstract of U.S. data on Alzheimer's disease.* Retrieved September 10, 2007, from http://www.alz.org/national/documents/Report_2007FactsAndFigures.pdf

Beach, S. R., Schulz, R., Williamson, G. M., Miller, L. S., Weiner, M. F., & Lance, C. E. (2005). Risk factors for potentially harmful informal caregiver behavior. *Journal of the American Geriatric Society, 53,* 255–261.

Beach, S. R., Schulz, R., Yee, J. L., & Jackson, S. (2000). Negative and positive health effects of caring for a disabled spouse: Longitudinal findings from the caregiver health effects study. *Psychology and Aging, 15,* 259–271.

Burns, R., Nichols, L. O., Martindale-Adams, J., Graney, M. J., & Lummus, A. (2003). Primary care interventions for dementia caregivers: 2-year outcomes from the REACH study. *Gerontologist, 43,* 547–555.

Cohen-Mansfield, J. (1995). Stress in nursing home staff: A review and a theoretical model. *Journal of Applied Gerontology, 14*(4), 444–466.

Cohen-Mansfield, J. (1997). Turnover among nursing home staff. *Nursing Management, 28*(5), 59–64.

Covinsky, K. E., Newcomer, R., Fox, P., Wood, J., Sands, L., Dane, K., & Yaffe, K. (2003). Patient and caregiver characteristics associated with depression in caregivers of patients with dementia. *Journal of General Internal Medicine, 18,* 1006–1114.

D'Eramo, A. L., Papp, K. K., & Rose, J. H. (2001). A program on complementary therapies for long-term care nursing assistants. *Geriatric Nursing, 22*(4), 201–207.

Dunn, L. A., Rout, U., Carson, J., & Ritter, S. A. (1994). Occupational stress amongst care staff working in nursing homes: An empirical investigation. *Journal of Clinical Nursing, 3*(3), 177–183.

Family Caregiver Alliance. (2001). *Fact Sheet: Side-by-Side Comparison of Family Caregiver Prevalence Studies.* Retrieved on September 14, 2007, from www.caregiver.org/caregiver/jsp/content/pdfs/fs_caregiver_stats_side_by_side.pdf

Feinberg, L. F., & Newman, S. L. (2006). A study of 10 states since passage of the National Family Caregiver Support Program: Policies, perceptions, and program development. *The Gerontologist, 46,* 344–356.

Goodman, C. R., Zarit, S. H., & Steiner, V. L. (1997). Personal orientation as a predictor of caregiver strain. *Aging & Mental Health, 1*(2), 149–157.

Kabat-Zinn, J. (1996). Mindfulness meditation, what it is, what it isn't and its role in healthcare and medicine. In Y. Haruki, Y. Ishii, & M. Suzuki (Eds.), pp. 161–170, *Comparative and Psychological Study on Meditation.* Delft, Netherlands: Eburon.

LeRoy, A. (2007). *Exhaustion, anger of caregiving get a name.* Retrieved September 4, 2007, from http://www.cnn.com/2007/HEALTH/conditions/08/13/caregiver.syndrome/index.html?eref=rss_health

López, J., Crespo, M., & Zarit, S. H. (2007). Assessment of the efficacy of a stress management program for informal caregivers of dependent older adults. *The Gerontologist, 47*(2), 205–214.

Minor, H. G., Carlson, L. E., Mackenzie, M. J., & Zernicke, K. (2006). Evaluation of a Mindfulness Based Stress Reduction (MBSR) program for caregivers of children with chronic conditions. *Social Work in Health Care, 43*(1), 91–109.

Mittelman, M. (2005, November). Taking care of the caregivers. *Current Opinion in Psychiatry, 18*(6), 633–639.

Mittelman, M. S., Roth, D. L., Coon, D. W., & Haley, W. E. (2004). Sustained benefit of supportive intervention for depressive symptoms in caregivers of patients with Alzheimer's disease. *American Journal of Psychiatry, 161*, 850–856.

Nursing home aides experience increase in serious injuries. *Monthly Labor Review Online, 113*(2). Retrieved September 10, 2007, from http://www.bls.gov/opub/mlr/1990/02/art4exc.htm

Pekkarinen, L., Sinervo, T., Perälä, M.-L., & Elovainio, M. (2004). Personick, M. E. (1990). Work stressors and the quality of life in long-term care units. *The Gerontologist, 44*(5), 633–643.

Personick, M. E. (1990). Nursing home aides experience increase in serious injuries. *Monthly Labor Review, 113*.

Pinquart, M., & Sörensen, S. (2003). Associations of stressors and uplifts of caregiving with caregiver burden and depressive mood: A meta-analysis. *The Journals of Gerontology Series B: Psychological Sciences and Social Sciences, 58*, 112–128.

Schenström, A., Rönnberg, S., & Bodlund, O. (2006). Mindfulness-based cognitive attitude training for primary care staff: A pilot study. *Complementary Health Practice Review, 11*(3), 144–152.

Schultz, R., & Beach, S. R. (1999). Caregiving as a risk factor for mortality: The Caregiver Health Effects Study. *Journal of the American Medical Association, 282*, 2215–2219.

Schulz, R., Belle, S., Czaja, S., McGinnis, K., Stevens, A., & Zhang, S. (2004). Long-term care placement of dementia patients and caregiver health and well-being. *Journal of the American Medical Association, 292*(8), 961–967.

Schulz, R., & Martire, L. M. (2004). Family caregiving of persons with dementia: Prevalence, health effects, and support strategies. *American Journal of Geriatric Psychiatry, 12*, 240–249.

Schulz, R., O'Brien, A. T., Bookwals, J., & Fleissner, K. (1995). Psychiatric and physical morbidity effects of dementia caregiving: Prevalence, correlates, and causes. *The Gerontologist, 35*, 771–791.

Schulz, R., O'Brien, A., Czaja, S., Ory, M., Norris, R., Martire, L. M., Belle, S. H., Burgio, L., Gitlin, L., Coon, D., Burns, S. H., Gallagher-Thompson, D., & Stevens, A. (2002). Dementia caregiver intervention research: In search of clinical significance. *The Gerontologist, 42*, 589–602.

Singh, N. N., Lancioni, G. E., Winton, A. S. W., Wahler, R. G., Singh, J., & Sage, M. (2004). Mindful caregiving increases happiness among individuals with profound multiple disabilities. *Research in Developmental Disabilities: A Multidisciplinary Journal, 25*(2), 207–218.

Stone, R. (2001, October). *Long term care workforce shortages: Impact on families.* Policy Brief No. 3. Commissioned for *Who will provide care? Emerging issues for state policymakers*. Funded by The Robert Wood Johnson Foundation. Retrieved September 8, 2007, from http://www.betterjobsbettercare.org/content/docs/LTC_Workforce_Shortages.pdf

Stone, R. I., & Wiener, J. M. (2001, October 26). *Who will care for us? Addressing the long-term care workforce crisis.* Retrieved September 4, 2007, from http://www.urban.org/url.cfm?ID=310304

Tabak, N., Ehrenfeld, M., & Alpert, R. (1997). Feelings of anger among caregivers of patients with Alzheimer's disease. *International Journal of Nursing Practice, 3*(2), 84–88.

Thomas, W. H. (2002, October). *& Thou Shalt Honor.* Retrieved September 14, 2007, from http://www.pbs.org/thoushalthonor/eden/index.html

Toseland, R. W. (1995). *Group work with the elderly and family caregivers.* New York: Springer.

Vitaliano, P. P., Scanlan, J. M., Krenz, C., & Fujtmoto, W. (1996). Insulin and glucose: Relationships with hassles, anger, and hostility in nondiabetic older adults. *Psychosomatic Medicine, 58,* 489–499.

Vitaliano, P. P., Zhang, J., & Scanlan, J. M. (2003). Is caregiving hazardous to one's physical health? A meta-analysis. *Psychological Bulletin, 129*(6), 946–972.

Waelde, L. C., Thompson, L., & Gallagher-Thompson, D. (2004). A pilot study of a yoga and meditation intervention for dementia caregiver stress. *Journal of Clinical Psychology, 60*(6), 677–687.

Wolff, J. L., & Kasper, J. D. (2006). Caregivers of frail elders: Updating a national profile. *The Gerontologist, 46,* 344–356.

Yates, M. E., Tennstedt, S., & Chang, B. H. (1999). Contributors to and mediators of psychological well-being for informal caregivers. *The Journals of Gerontology Series B: Psychological Sciences and Social Sciences, 54*(1), 12–22.

Zimmerman, S., Williams, C. S., Reed, P. S., Boustani, M., Preisser, J. S., Heck, E., & Sloane, P. D. (2005). Attitudes, stress, and satisfaction of staff who care for residents with dementia. *The Gerontologist, 45,* 96–105.

CHAPTER 10

Riding the Waves:
Mindfulness-Based Elder Care
for Informal Caregivers

ONE CAREGIVER'S STORY

Mr. R was a 92-year-old man whose wife of 65 years was admitted to a nursing home. The Rs were childless, and all other relatives were deceased. Although it was unclear if Mrs. R still recognized her husband, he visited daily, staying from before lunch until after supper. The Rs had spent their savings on Mrs R's home care before she was admitted to the nursing home, and Mr. R took a long bus ride for his daily visit. One day there was a severe blizzard. The previous day, staff had encouraged Mr. R to stay at home, but he appeared at the nursing home and stayed all day. It was dark by late afternoon; the snow was falling heavily; and Mr. R. was going out the door. After much encouragement, Mr. R did accept transportation provided by the facility. I watched him leave with trepidation and was struck by his need to visit daily.

Nursing home workers often comment that they are more concerned about the family, friends, and other unpaid informal caregivers than the residents they visit. Caregivers, whether family, significant others, or friends of the frail elders are frequently at risk for their own stress-related problems. Caregivers often focus on the needs of the care recipient to the neglect of their own health. Many are old and may suffer from their own health problems, compounded by the stress of caregiving. Caregiver literature and interventions generally focus on community caregivers, even though nonprofessional caregivers for nursing home residents are also at risk. These caregivers may find themselves mentally preoccupied with the responsibility of caring for their friend or family member even when not providing direct care or visiting. Publicity or reports of poor care at nursing homes can add to this sense of guilt, responsibility, and burden. Caregivers of nursing home residents often feel excluded from discussions on general caregiving issues. This omission can make it harder to acknowledge their need.

Offering mindfulness programs for informal caregivers of frail elders is most helpful when modifications made the format allow for time constraints and more targeted the discussion on caregiving. In my experience, informal caregivers appreciate time-limited, psychoeducational groups that offer both skills and support. A psychoeducational group that offers skills in stress reduction is especially appropriate for a highly stressed population, and it is also reflected in the research (López, Crespo, & Zarit, 2007).

Informal caregivers often report being stressed or having stress-related health problems. Therefore, I was surprised when the groups offered to caregivers of a 514-bed nursing home were not in high demand. Most caregivers find it difficult to justify taking care of themselves, despite reports of the need. Though their family member or friend is now in the nursing home, they may still feel time constraints from busy lives. It may be helpful to remind caregivers that they can better care for others if they care for themselves first. This chapter discusses Mindfulness-Based Elder Care groups, held in a nursing home, for caregivers of nursing home residents.

Caregiver group members are recruited through public postings, mailings, and referrals from nursing home staff. Participants are interviewed in advance to ensure that the course will not take the place of individual therapy, when needed. The intake interview may also be a good time to review the expectations and to ask participants to make an initial commitment to practice and attend the group. In my experience, the benefits reaped from this course are proportionate to the dedication to practice outside of the group. I state this up front in my initial interviews and encourage commitment throughout the course.

Caregiver participants usually self-identify as experiencing physical and emotional problems. The groups I will discuss in this chapter suggest the general norms of caregivers. Their age ranges from 45–80; they are female; and are siblings, daughters, spouses, and even ex-wives. Groups are 1 1/2 hours long, and no all-day session was offered. The courses are held in the nursing home where the care receiver resides.

> F said that she was learning to enjoy her time with her father now that he is in the nursing home, but felt she was still suffering from the effects of an extended period of caregiving in the community. Right now, she reminds herself that her father is cared for, and she can relax, but worrying has become a habit.

OVERVIEW OF CLASS

In caregiver groups, the variety of techniques taught includes deep breathing, visualization, gentle yoga, and mindfulness. Participants practice the skills in the group and between sessions, with the help of instructions on a CD provided. Each week a new practice is taught or reviewed. After the first session, each group begins with a few moments of silent sitting. This time becomes longer each week. A discussion of skills from the previous weeks follows, with time provided for any thoughts or concerns about them and any questions. The discussion focuses on learning to look at events differently and how the participants can use what they learned in their daily lives. Following the discussion, a new technique is presented or reviewed and practiced. The group ends with another period of silent sitting. At the conclusion, the next week's homework is discussed, handouts reinforcing the practice are distributed, and practice suggestions are offered. The caregiver group is very experiential and personal, evoking powerful responses from the participants.

> V said that her husband's roommate died this week. She became tearful and talked about how this was rehearsal for what she would be dealing with someday. She talked about other residents and the roommate's family. She became tearful again and said that having a family member in the nursing home brought one face to face with life's challenges.

Caregivers often respond positively to the mindfulness group and say they benefit from and use the skills to make positive changes in their lives. As stated above, changes are made to the model to accommodate the schedules of the participants and their physical stamina. Ongoing encouragement is also helpful. If a participant misses a session, I call and send the handouts and homework. That is also a good time to check on their practice and answer any questions. Caregivers let me know they appreciate this support and find it easier to return to the group and to keep up. Initially tapes made by other mindfulness instructors were used for the practice tapes. In class, however, group members were accustomed to my voice and asked me if I could tape it. The voice of a known instructor can provide continuity and support. New technology makes it easier to record ourselves and to make CDs; it is worth the effort.

INTRODUCTIONS

Caregivers frequently focus on their own family member when visiting, and do not connect with the natural support system of other visiting caregivers. In addition, their schedules may vary, and caregivers with much in common may not cross paths. Introducing them to each other establishes the commonality of interests and support that comes from shared concerns. It is also helpful to establish the participant's previous experience with meditation and yoga. Often, we assume that an older person has not meditated or practiced yoga. In my experience this assumption is not true!

> Caregiver group participants shared a little about their circumstances and their expectations from the group. All members stated that they were feeling quite stressed and had multiple burdens. In addition to having family members at the nursing home, many had their own illnesses and other family problems or life stressors.

The introduction can also serve to describe the course as a place to learn stress reduction in a supportive, nonjudgmental atmosphere. Caregivers may have difficulty taking care of themselves. When they do take care of themselves, they may feel guilty or nervous. Feelings of guilt over being healthy or taking time away from the care recipient are common. Unlike traditional support groups, this group is primarily an opportunity to learn new ways of being and perceiving, as well as stress reduction skills experientially. In this context, many find themselves, and the caregiving experience, changed.

FORMAL PRACTICES

Diaphragmatic Breathing

To begin with, the diaphragmatic, three-part, deep belly breath is demonstrated and practiced. Participants often report it as the most utilized and helpful skill. This is followed with a breath awareness meditation, in which the breath is observed but not manipulated. The meditations are initially short, 5–10 minutes, and become increasingly longer as the course progresses. In the first session I explain that all future sessions will start with a period of silent sitting. Taking time out to just sit and focus awareness on the in breath and the out breath is an excellent way to begin the group. The quiet sitting establishes a tone of reflectiveness and shifts us from the busyness of our day. It also allows for latecomers to enter quietly. Following this practice, participants can engage in a more mindful discussion, paying full attention to what they choose to share, as well as fully listening to their peers. Throughout the group, we practice periods of quiet sitting, short and long, as needed to recenter the group members' focus.

Breath Awareness

In breath awareness, participants are asked to focus on their breath: the in breath and the out breath, without directing it in any particular way. It is helpful to identify one area to focus on, such as the nostrils or the area under the nostril, noticing the cool breath entering and the warm breath exiting; or the chest or the belly as they gently rise and fall.

> M said she enjoyed the breathing. She said the breathing helps her from reacting so quickly to events. When her grandkids bother her, she now takes a breath and finds she is not as angry as before the breath.

Meditation: Shifting From a Mode of Doing to a Mode of Being

> M reported that during the meditation, she began to think about her mother and to wonder if she was doing enough. Once this happened she was unable to let the thought go. Commenting on the meditation, she said, "It's not as easy as it sounds."

Often meditation looks easy until it is tried. When we first sit still and begin to observe our breath, we find ourselves pulled away again and again. Group members often need reminding that this is a new practice, and, like anything new that we try, it may take time to establish. Mindfulness teacher Jack Kornfeld, in *A Path With Heart* (1993), suggests adopting an attitude toward initial meditation practice similar to that of training a puppy. Owners of a new puppy understand that it takes time, patience, consistency, and love to train the dog. He suggests that we adopt this same attitude toward ourselves as we learn a challenging new practice. This attitude establishes intention and discipline, at the same time as kindness and self-compassion.

> S said that she wasn't sure she was being aware of the present moment because she felt "numb in her body." R said that she had previous experience in a yoga center where the music was louder, the incense stronger, and the lights lower. In the yoga center she had really relaxed, and she did not feel as relaxed this time.

New meditation practitioners may also have preconceptions of relaxation or expectations of stress reduction. Mindfulness offers a powerful practice in letting go of the "what ifs." Learning stress reduction may even feel stressful at times. Our minds will wander; it is our practice just to notice this, and return our attention to the object of our meditation. Mindfulness is not the same as relaxation, Kabat-Zinn (1994) reminds us. Relaxation is temporal. Relaxation is viewed as "successful," "curing" stress. Mindfulness is constantly present and timeless. Mindfulness heals, not necessarily cures. Relaxation may be a result of mindfulness practices, but it is not the intention. Mindfulness may also be stressful and challenging. Being present to emotions in our life, we fully engage with suffering, boredom, and joy. Being present in our body, we sit with pain, neutrality, and pleasure.

Meditation in Movement

Bodywork can be very helpful for caregivers. In quiet seated meditation practice, the mind may become very active. It is much harder to have a wandering mind while trying to balance on one foot or stretch the hamstrings! In addition, caregivers may not have many opportunities to exercise and to stretch. Physical exercise may hold many benefits for the mind, body, and soul. In caregiver courses exercises are integrated into every session. In mindful movement, I consider the back or spine: stretching it up and down, twisting it side to side, and curving it in and out. Participants are also reminded to listen to their own bodies and only to do what feels right to them.

> One woman talked about doing her exercises mindfully in her sister's room while visiting. Her sister has advanced dementia, but seemed calmed by this experience.

Exercises on the Floor

In caregiver groups, participants are encouraged to use mats and get down on the floor for yoga. I also offer the option of chair exercises for participants who have physical conditions that prevent them from getting down on the floor. In these cases, participants are advised to try floor exercises on their beds at home. Chairs are always available as well as mats, and instructions are modified for those in chairs. For example, stretching and twisting can be done seated or lying down.

Seated Exercises

Many caregivers spend time at desks, or seated for other reasons. Offering seated exercises can provide ways for caregivers to integrate stress reduction and bodywork into their busy schedules. Chair poses are included in Appendix A. Face and eye exercises may be helpful and also playful.

TRY THIS

Start with standing, centering. Imagine for a moment that you are a tree. Breathe, feel your feet on the ground, planted. Feel your body sway gently as the trees do in the wind. Bring your awareness to your whole body, standing. Feel your head in the sky, your feet on the ground, your body connecting heaven and earth. It may help to close your eyes. You may feel an impulse to move, but stay with the standing a little longer, explore the desire to move without needing to respond to it. See if you can feel your strength, rooted, planted into the ground. Trees are connected to the earth through their roots, and also reach to the sky, moving with the wind. Their strength comes from their roots and their flexibility.

Standing Poses

Most people spend time standing, either in line or waiting for transportation. In caregiver groups we also practice standing mindfully. We also practice balancing exercises, lifting first one foot and lowering it, then the other. The arms can go out to the side, or the hands can hold the back of a chair or the wall as needed.

Free Movement to Music

Free movement to music can provide not only exercise, but also emotional expression and release. Learning to tune into our bodies and expressing ourselves through movement can be liberating. If participants are uncomfortable, they can keep their eyes closed.

Walking Meditation

Caregivers in these groups live in a busy urban area, and the idea of walking without needing to get anywhere is novel. After practicing mindful walking, some participants observe it is easier to meditate while walking.

> N says that during the walking meditation she was able not to think about her husband, who is not eating. N has been considering a feeding tube. She says she thought about her husband all day at work and even during the group, but during the walking meditation, she could let go.

Caregivers often struggle with difficult decisions and life issues. Choosing a feeding tube may extend quantity of life, but not necessarily quality. On the other hand, if an elder is not eating, and a family member chooses not to place a feeding tube, the elder may not survive. Mindfulness practices may offer a way to find space and time in which to contemplate these decisions in a thoughtful way. In the walking meditation, N found this space.

INFORMAL PRACTICE

Informal mindfulness is being aware in any moment. In the caregiver group, an essential component is the discussion of the use of this practice, or paying attention, outside of class. Many mindfulness practices, like standing and walking, can also be done informally throughout the day.

M said she practiced standing meditation informally, in many places such as in the bank line, and she found it calming.

Sometimes, group members begin to notice their lives in new ways.

S said that she did not do the homework, but did notice when she was playing with her grandchild that she was able to forget everything else.

Eating Awareness

S said that she ate raisins all the time, but she usually gulped them down by the handful. She said this was the best raisin she ever ate. W said that when the raisin was in her mouth it became plump, and mentioned that often in cooking one plumps the raisins first.
N said that she was unable to eat slowly, but connected raisins with events from her past.

Each mindful experience offers rich lessons. Despite commonalities, caregivers may begin to observe that they experience life uniquely. They may notice how awareness changes us and our experience of life. They may notice that slowing down and paying attention can provide a new relationship with eating. Caregivers learn to consider bringing a similar awareness to other ordinary events in their lives.

DISCUSSION

Group discussion can offer an opportunity to explore thoughts that arise, answer questions, and discover the normalcy of many experiences. It is often helpful to discourage intellectual discussions and to stay with the practice and the participants' experience of it. Words that often come up are *try* and *should*. When this happens, it can be helpful to remind caregivers of the mindfulness principle of being with what *is*.

Group members anecdotally report changes in their lives in large and small ways.

> K said that she had noticed a subtle change in her need to be busy. That she felt more okay about not "taking on" so much. S said that she had a hard week but now could relax. B said she hadn't thought about it, but now she noticed that she had not fought with her daughter all week, and this was different. She thinks it might have something to do with her being able to let things go more easily. She also said that she really looks forward to the group. A said she had moved recently, and it was hard, but when she needed to, she would lie down and breathe, and it would refresh her.

Mindfulness courses offer a range of tools and encourage participants to fully experience their lives. The tools may be helpful in increasing present moment awareness of pleasure and may also increase awareness of other strong feelings, including annoyance or boredom.

> We practiced the standing and walking meditations. I noticed that people stopped walking after 5 minutes. Some people had physical difficulty, but everyone sat down. We discussed people's reaction to the walking meditation. S and R said they found walking slowly intolerable. They walked to get someplace and could not "just" walk. M and T said they usually had trouble walking and yet had found the slow walking to be less painful and more pleasurable.

Use of Imagery and Poetry

In mindfulness groups, poetry and imagery can provide an alternative way of conveying the principles. Appendix F includes references to poets and writers often aligned with mindfulness practices. For some caregivers, the images help deepen understanding. A chapter from Kabat-Zinn's *Wherever You Go, There You Are* (1994), titled "You Can't Stop the Waves, but You Can Learn to Surf," resonated with one caregiver, who, in her feedback at the end of the course, said:

I feel less anxious about stresses than I formerly did. I think about "riding the waves" instead of getting anxious about them or "fighting" the waves. I feel less responsible for my husband's well-being.

Guided Imagery or Visualization

Guided imagery and visualization encompass a large range of practices. In the context of mindfulness practice, visualization is not wishing for things to be different. It may provide a metaphor for understanding concepts (Kabat-Zinn, 1990). One practice some find helpful is connecting with an inner guide. Based on Gawain's (1991) visualizations, I incorporated this practice into one caregiver group. Caregivers may feel their own lives are hijacked and may lose personal direction when consumed with caregiving. This practice proved helpful in reconnecting them to their deeper selves.

I asked members to sit quietly, then, imagine a place where they felt comfortable. It is helpful in guided imagery to use all the senses, so the group was encouraged to imagine smells, sounds, and touch, as well as sight. They could imagine a place in nature or a place inside. When they were comfortable, I asked them to imagine a guide coming to them. This guide could take any form, be human or animal. Participants were asked to engage with the guide and to listen (Gawain, 1991).

> After the visualization, caregivers reported their experiences. S found herself in a room that was uncomfortable, but then moved to a room that she felt good in. K found herself in several places that she could vividly imagine, even though she said she had no imagination. A said she could imagine the inner guide and that "she no longer felt she had to be alone ever again." She felt as though the guide were a part of herself, an alter ego.

In this exercise, participants used their imagination to listen deeply to their inner wisdom.

The Role of Perception

In group discussions, caregiver group members are encouraged to look at their lives differently. The experience of caregiving can be stressful, but also an opportunity to deepen the relationship between caregiver and care provider. Mindfulness practice often brings an awareness to practitioners of greater options in their lives. Caregivers participating in these mindfulness groups often reported increased pleasure in the caregiving experience. They still experienced challenges and stress, and they also found increasing moments in which they could be *present*.

> K sits in the nursing home's garden with her mother. She is aware of the flowers in bloom and the warm day. She also is aware that she is sharing this with her mother. B is slowed down by foot surgery. She notices the sky and trees and feels gratitude. T said her dog had an accident on the rug and she cleaned it up mindfully, and M told how her husband took a wrong turn, and she could stay with her breath.

Pleasant and Unpleasant Events

The pleasant and unpleasant events calendar is a daily record participants are asked to keep. On it, they note events as they occur and feelings, physical sensations, and thoughts associated with these events. This practice proved useful for some in the caregiver classes. (The pleasant/unpleasant events calendar is described in detail in Kabat-Zinn [1990], pp. 142–143, 446–449.)

> K said that she had found the pleasant events calendar helpful. She said that her father is rapidly declining, and she had been tracking the positive interactions and shared times. It had helped her enjoy the time with her father and not just focus on his decline.

Group Experience

Many group members report that the group experience is very important. Group members supported and encouraged each other.

> S said she appreciated the work and energy that was put into the group. She said that the energy that was shared in the group had enabled her to carry the work into her own life.
> She also commented that she found it different to meditate with the group. Others agreed that the meditation experience was different in the group.

Many find meditating with others is supportive and connecting. Also, initially, instruction and guidance may be important. At the same time, I encourage home practice, using CDs as needed, to establish an ongoing foundation of personal practice.

Anger and Forgiveness

Caregiving can engender many feelings, and the feelings themselves may bring further distress and shame. Anger is one common response to the overwhelming and demanding aspects of caregiving. In caregiver groups, I have found it to be helpful to discuss anger, as well as other strong feelings, as part of mindfulness practice. These groups are not psychotherapeutically oriented; the discussion usually focuses on a body awareness of anger. One helpful exercise is the Anger Continuum (B. Roth, personal communication, April 29, 2003). This exercise begins by asking the participants to close their eyes and remember a time that they were angry. Participants are asked what they noticed—where they felt it in their bodies. After we have briefly discussed this experience, participants describe anger in all its variations. The words that arise may be *rage, fury, irritation, distress, annoyance*. If needed, I add words to the discussion. These words are written on 8-1/2 by 11 sheets of paper. When enough words have been generated, I place them in a line on the wall, ranging from the mildest— perhaps annoyance—to the strongest—perhaps rage. We observe that anger holds a range of feelings. When we become more aware of the shades of our feelings by noticing them in our bodies, we may be able take appropriate action when the feelings are still mild rather than when they are raging and more difficult to control.

> F said that when she is angry, she can "do" something. Underneath the anger, she feels sadness—sad that there is no one to be angry at, nothing to do. Her mother is unhappy here [at the nursing home], and she feels like she needs to fix this. Others suggest that she cannot change her mother. T talks about an outburst of anger toward her father.

The discussion is often followed with a forgiveness meditation. (A suggested script of this meditation is available in Appendix B.) In the forgiveness meditation, participants can begin by forgiving themselves, and then, if comfortable, forgive others. Many caregivers find the practice of forgiving themselves to be powerfully healing. Despite the tremendous responsibilities carried, caregivers often feel they are not doing enough or not doing it correctly.

> One caregiver had been taking care of her husband for 10 years following a stroke. Their happy retirement plans were destroyed. Although she took good care of her spouse, in the mindfulness class, she discovered how angry she was while providing the care. She now takes care of herself, as well as him, differently by going to exercise classes and practicing mindfulness (J. Vega, personal communication, August 29, 2007).

Homework

Homework is regularly assigned. In general, group members are asked to continue informal and formal skills discussed and experienced in sessions. Setting aside time each day for meditation or yoga may establish a routine that, by the end of a course, becomes a foundation for ongoing practice. I suggest to group members that they try practicing at different times and places, noting which locations and times work best. Informally, participants are asked to eat mindfully, practice the deep breathing throughout the day, and bring mindful attention to regular activities such as brushing teeth and washing dishes.

In the group, we bring our attention not only to the directed activities or discussion, but also to the transitions. Sometimes, participants are asked to notice transitions in their lives, whether walking from one place to another, moving from one activity to another, waiting in line or for transportation. For those with busy lives, these times may feel wasted or frustrating. It is also a precious time to be awake and present. They can be a chance to practice mindfulness, observing sensations, feelings, and thoughts that arise in these "in-between" moments.

> This week, group members report not doing formal homework but noticing how the practice has become part of their lives. B commented that while waiting 1-1/2 hours for an appointment, she felt less angry and took the opportunity to breathe, relax, and meditate. J reported that in a cab she felt herself getting stressed because she was late. She noticed it and allowed herself to let it go. J reported that the only time she has to slow down is when she walks her dogs. She walks them slowly, observing nature.

Group participants are asked to make a commitment to practicing the skills learned in class on a regular basis. For the instructor and participants, however, there is a fine line between commitment and compassion. For caregivers who are already feeling overwhelmed and self-critical, the best practice may be self-compassion. For myself, I learn to let go, over and over, of the outcomes.

> F said she was not able to practice for no particular reason; she just seemed to put it off. This sparked a huge discussion. T stated that she was a "meditation drop out." All nodded, as if they felt the same way.

Practicing meditation is challenging and also a great opportunity to practice kindness to ourselves. In caregiver groups, it is helpful to emphasize practicing with discipline and also practicing with kindness. If caregivers cannot practice the full amount of time, it may be beneficial to suggest that they practice a short meditation, gradually stretching the limits.

ENDINGS AND ONGOING PRACTICE

As the course ends, members are asked to consider their ongoing practice: what has been helpful, what can they realistically continue? Many feel that ongoing support would be helpful, and I make referrals to local meditation and yoga resources.

Letter to Self

In the caregiver mindfulness groups, the skills we learn are signs pointing to what we know already or to discovering new things about ourselves. We give ourselves time to remember and explore. In the last session, I ask group members to take a few moments during meditation to consider what they had remembered or learned about themselves in the course. I give members note cards and ask them to write a letter to themselves. No one else will read it. What would they want to remind themselves of in the future? When the card is finished, they put it in a self-addressed envelope and seal it. I will send it to them in a month.

Postgroup

Changes reported are ongoing and often subtle.

> One month after the group's ending, A reports she had to go out West for her uncle's funeral. It was the first time she was away from her sister. She thought it would be difficult to be away, but noticed that she felt more relaxed than she anticipated. She asked if that was a mindful experience.

CAREGIVER MINDFULNESS GROUP RESEARCH

In 1996, a 10-week, 1 1/2–hour mindfulness group was offered for family and significant others of nursing home residents. The members consisted of 8 caregivers, with an age range of 60–85 years. All were female; some were daughters, spouses, ex-spouses, or siblings. All participants were self-identified as experiencing physical and emotional problems. In the caregiver group, we practiced deep breathing, visualization, gentle yoga, and mindfulness. Participants were encouraged to practice between sessions with the help of taped instructions. After the course, members were asked to fill out a brief open-ended questionnaire about their experiences. Anecdotal reports were positive, with most caregivers reporting a decrease in stress and somatic complaints as well as an increased satisfaction in the caregiver role. One caregiver stated, "There are things I learned in this group that I can—and will—apply and live with the rest of my life."

In 2005, an 8-week MBSR course was offered for informal caregivers of nursing home residents as part of a research study. Caregivers who participated in the study were over age 18 and spent more than 20 hours per week caring, or supervising care for, a family member or friend. Nine women, mostly daughters, aged 48 to 73, participated in seven or more MBSR groups. Self-report measures of depression, anxiety, stress, grief, burden, and mindfulness were obtained at study entry, after 8 weeks of MBSR training, and 1 month following completion of the MBSR program. Results showed medium-effect-size estimates for reduction in stress and burden during active treatment, persisting 4 weeks following completion of the intervention. Self-reported depression, anxiety, grief, and perceived stress and burden decreased during the 8-week intervention with further reduction demonstrated after a 4-week follow-up in all measures except depression. No change in measure over time was statistically significant, however. Qualitatively, participants reported personal benefits from the training and continued use of the acquired skills (Epstein-Lubow, McBee, & Miller, 2007).

SUMMARY

In mindfulness groups, members become increasingly aware of their daily activities and are able to experience their lives more fully. In stressful situations, they state that they are able to respond more thoughtfully and less reactively. They are able to focus on the positive and enjoy the moment more rather than focusing on the future or the past. Many use the techniques to help with sleeping problems. Also, the progress of individual members appears to inspire other members as the group's cohesiveness grows. All members note simple but powerful changes in their quality of life.

> V said that she experienced pleasure, but that it was tinged with sadness sometimes when she thought that her husband was not there to share it. Nevertheless, she could allow herself to feel pleasure at times.

REFERENCES

Epstein-Lubow, G., McBee, L., & Miller, I. W. (2007). *Mindful caregiving and the perception of burden in family members of frail elderly.* Poster presentation. Center for Mindfulness in Medicine, Healthcare and Society, 2007 Annual Conference, Worcester, MA.

Gawain, S. (1991). *Meditations: Creative visualization and meditation exercises to enrich your life.* Novato, CA: Nataraj.

Kabat-Zinn, J. (1990). *Full catastrophe living: Using the wisdom of your body and mind to face stress, pain and illness.* New York: Dell.

Kabat-Zinn, J. (1994). *Wherever you go, there you are: Mindfulness meditation in everyday life.* New York: Hyperion.

Kornfield, J. (1993). *A path with heart: A guide through the perils and promises of spiritual life.* New York: Bantam.

López, J., Crespo, M., & Zarit, S. H. (2007). Assessment of the efficacy of a stress management program for informal caregivers of dependent older adults. *The Gerontologist, 47*(2), 205–214.

CHAPTER 11

Learning to Take Care of Myself: A 7-Week Mindfulness-Based Elder Care Course

I'm learning to take time for myself with all my body parts.

—Staff caregiver

The ideal offering for professional caregivers is an 8-week MBSR course with ongoing support. A substantial commitment is required for a traditional MBSR program, however. Nursing home and hospital staff can only be away from their responsibilities for brief periods, and staff "backfill," or replacements, are crucial to offering uninterrupted classes with regular attendance.

A 7-week, 1-hour MBEC course was offered to approximately 100 staff members, supported in part by a grant from the United Hospital Fund of New York. The grant targeted caregivers of palliative care patients in the nursing home. I and/or a certified yoga teacher taught the classes. This chapter details the highlights of this course and offers suggestions and recommendations for similar programs.

OVERVIEW OF CAREGIVER COURSE

Class Participants

MBEC course participants were recruited from two preselected 38-bed units in a large urban facility. This staff was chosen because the pace and stress level for these units was high. Staff were released from their assignments to attend the course, but not mandated to attend. Sharing the experience was helpful in several ways. The participants concurred that their work environment was stressful. They found it beneficial to have a dedicated time and place to share these feelings and to learn new ways to cope with them. Staff members began to know each other as individuals, outside of their usual role or profession. They came to see each other as colleagues and to view one another in new ways. And participants reinforced the skills outside of the group, encouraging each other to take a break and breathe or eat mindfully. Daytime course participants were doctors, rehab therapists, social workers, dieticians, therapeutic recreation workers, nurses, nursing assistants, and housekeepers. Evening and night participants were nursing assistants and nurses.

Certain themes emerged in working with these professional caregivers. The majority of participants were entry-level workers, mostly nursing assistants, and a few housekeeping staff. They provide the most difficult and poorly paid care and are overwhelmingly represented by minorities and new immigrants. Low levels of socioeconomic status and their accompanying stressors are typical. Language or educational level may be a consideration, too. The profile of this cohort resembles the population described by Roth and Calle-Mesa (2006), as do the practical applications and considerations. In their chapter "Mindfulness-Based Stress Reduction (MBSR) with Spanish- and English-speaking inner-city medical patients," these authors summarize the connections among minority status, low socioeconomic status (SES), health, and stress, as well as the benefits of MBSR for this population.

Recruitment

Course members were recruited in more than one way. Informational flyers and sign-up sheets were on the unit. What proved to be the most effective, however, were one-to-one conversations with the staff. While this nursing home staff regularly reported being stressed, we noted that direct care workers were reluctant to sign up for a stress reduction course. Previous experience with in-service classes in the nursing home may have partially accounted for this reluctance. Most classes offered for direct care staff are mandatory and oriented toward patient care or regulatory compliance. These caregivers may justifiably view job-related classes as adding to their workload without improving their working conditions. Some caregivers may have limited education or limited English. A class may be intimidating. One caregiver, who was reluctant to sign up for the course, finally asked me if there would be a test!

We found it helpful to speak to caregivers individually or in small groups. We also offered short, introductory sessions on the unit, demonstrating what would be taught in the course. It was especially effective to offer hand massages to the caregivers. While providing the hand massage to the staff member, we could describe the course and allow the potential participant to get to know us a little better. We also found a trusted "leader" from the unit as an advocate. One of the doctors was a meditation practitioner, and she encouraged staff, whom she knew well, to attend.

There was no intake interview of staff for these groups; the courses were open to all who wished to attend. It was especially important, therefore, for instructors to be attentive to the participants' responses to the practices. Meditation and mindfulness may evoke or uncover strong feelings or repressed events. We had referrals for low-cost or sliding-scale therapy available and would speak with participants individually, as needed.

COURSE HIGHLIGHTS

Course Format

Sessions were 1 hour, but since they were held off the unit in a remote location, realistically, they were often 45 minutes. We provided journals and CDs, as well as weekly handouts. (Roth and Calle-Mesa [2006] did not provide handouts due to educational and language difficulties.) Staff were encouraged to participate in all sessions and asked to do practice homework. Sessions began with a time of quiet sitting; sometimes, guided meditations, sometimes, silence. As the course progressed, the sitting time became longer. We also incorporated movement and stretching into each session. In between, the yoga teacher was available on the units to provide support, mini sessions, instruction, and encouragement.

The MBEC for staff course focused on skills that would benefit both the caregiver and the care receiver. The six sessions were as follows:

1. Introduction to mindfulness, eating awareness exercise, deep breathing, body scan.
2. Meditation and aromatherapy.
3. Gentle yoga.
4. Guided imagery.
5. Communication and ways of perceiving.
6. Hand massage.
7. Palliative care, applications of CAM to resident care.

Introduction

The introduction was an opportunity to clarify expectations and provide encouragement for participants. This course was very different from those previously experienced by these participants. In the caregiver MBEC course, the learning was experiential, there were no wrong answers, and each individual's participation was valued. The instructor's nonjudgmental and supportive presence was significant for hesitant members. Roth and Calle-Mesa recount the statement of one despairing participant: "At that first meeting I trusted you immediately. I felt a glimmer of hope that this program might help me, even a little" (2006, p. 269). We also found it to be helpful to ask people in the course how they currently cope with stress. Sharing this information helped us to know where to begin and also to build the beginnings of camaraderie, since many people found they were coping in similar ways.

Deep Breathing

The deep breathing was so soul searching and relaxing. [It] make[s] me more aware of myself.

Learning to take deep, slow breaths is one mind-body intervention that may reduce our stress. Staff caregivers are often in stressful or crisis situations, responding to resident needs and behaviors as well as family requests and demands. At the same time, staff cope with ongoing paperwork and care provision responsibilities. When stressed, one way our bodies may respond is to breathe more rapidly and shallowly. Practiced regularly, deep breathing may become instinctive.

Meditation

I'm learning I can take just a few minutes out of my day to find that centeredness within myself by simply breathing and quieting my mind.

Most members of the caregiver group had no previous experience with meditation, and yet, many found it helpful and important in their lives. While finding time for extended formal practice was not available to most, just sitting quietly for a few minutes was restorative. We practiced meditation in all sessions and encouraged a home practice with CDs for guidance.

Yoga

I'm pretty flexible for my age. I like myself.

In this class we integrated movement into every session. In addition to yoga on the mat, we practiced chair-seated yoga, standing yoga, and wall yoga. While some participants had previous yoga experience, many had no formal exercise or bodywork training. Caregiving can be extremely, physically demanding. For many, learning to move mindfully and listen to their bodies was a new experience. Yoga provides exercise and movement, but also an increased body awareness that can be incorporated into all of our movements—or stillness.

Midway Review

When the course was half over, we asked participants to complete a midway review. It proved to be useful for both participants and instructors. We used a one-page written questionnaire to ascertain how the course was going for the staff members. The questions focused on their progress, problems, and concerns, and their ability to practice. We adjusted our teaching for the remaining sessions based on these responses. Some quieter participants could take this opportunity to share their opinions. Each course is unique, and there is always something new to learn! In addition, the questionnaire can serve the members as a motivator and reminder that the course time is limited. Participants can also self-assess based on the questions and consider how they want to best use their time and the practices. A copy of the Midway Review is available in Appendix E.

The Anger Continuum and Forgiveness Meditation

The course curriculum was significantly altered based on the instructors' observations of the staff's needs. During the initial sessions, staff expressed considerable anger at the workload expectations and the perceived lack of management responsiveness to their needs and input. Based on this information, we felt a session on anger would be an important aspect of this group. Roth and Calle-Mesa (2006) also report finding this discussion important, and the chapter's first author developed the Anger Continuum (Roth, personal communications, April 29, 2003; September 14, 2007). As described in Chapter 10, the Anger Continuum is an exercise that identifies the range of emotions associated with this emotion as well as the physical symptoms.

We introduced the Anger Continuum in session five. Staff participants may previously have had the perception that all classes are focused on improving patient care. At this point in the course, participants had begun to report the benefits of mindfulness practice for themselves. There was increased trust in the teachers and openness in the discussion. Although group members were clear that they were angry, they found the Anger Continuum discussion enlightening. The physical impact of anger was explored in meditation and discussion. Participants were able to link feelings of anger with tightness, pain, or distress in specific areas of their bodies. The Anger Continuum discussion provided insight into the range of feelings evoked by this powerful emotion. Most staff participants appreciated learning to identify earlier signals of anger, such as irritation and frustration, and benefited from discussions on responding to early physical signals.

Learning the early physical and mental distress signals of anger, or any strong emotion, is often valuable information. It may be more helpful if we know ways of appropriately coping with situations we may not be able to change. At this time, it is beneficial to ask participants to review what they are learning in class. We talked about deep breathing, taking a time out, or S.T.O.P. (see Chapter 5) when in crisis. Physical movement can often diffuse anger. We also suggested that a regular practice of the skills taught in the course might assist in shifting how participants would respond to crises in the long run.

> If your house is on fire, the most urgent thing to do is go back and try to put out the fire, not to run after the person you believe to be the arsonist. If you run after the person you suspect has burned your house, your house will burn down while you are chasing him or her. That is not wise. You must go back and put out the fire. So when you are angry, if you continue to interact with the other person, if you try to punish him or her, you are acting exactly like someone who runs after the arsonist while everything goes up in flames. (Nhat Hanh, 2001, p. 24)

One way of "putting out the flames" is to do a forgiveness meditation. This practice can follow the Anger Continuum, as we did, or provide a theme for a separate session (Roth, personal communication, September 14, 2007). It is important to clarify that forgiveness is actively taking care of our selves. We emphasized that forgiveness is not passively condoning thoughts and actions. The forgiveness meditation is a way of letting go of anger that may hurt us more than anyone else. We also underlined that participants need only do what is comfortable for them, starting with self-forgiveness. If caregivers felt comfortable forgiving others, they could include it in their meditation. We also point out that we do not have to share the forgiveness meditation with others, including those forgiven. The sessions on anger and forgiveness engendered lively discussions and new insights for staff.

> [I am learning] to keep myself calm and relax by closing my eyes, taking a deep breath.

Homework

In the midway review, many staff members reported that they were taking time to practice what we were learning in the course regularly (from daily to twice a week). Others, however, complained of being too busy and asked for continued structured sessions.

> I wish I could have the session more often. I'd like to do the exercises more often at home, but just can't seem to find the time.
> It has been difficult—I feel so busy all the time.

This situation may be realistic since some staff held two jobs, and others had multiple responsibilities outside of work.

DISCUSSION

Staff Response

Participants in the course responded positively to the practices. The Midway Review elicited these responses among others:

> This course is very important to me; it helps me to relax myself even for a few moments.
> It has brought a different perspective in my viewing of my body awareness.

In addition to positive qualitative reports, it was noted that staff retention on the units that participated in the course was 100% compared to other units and to these same units in other years.

The response to the sessions could be surprisingly positive at times. Night staff (the 11:30 p.m.–7:30 a.m. shift) often were delighted that they were included in the program. Both instructors had the sense that most of the staff participants would not have been exposed to mindfulness, meditation, or yoga otherwise, and some expressed sincere and heartfelt gratitude for the experience. Or as one nursing assistant said, "You go girls!"

Instructor Criteria

In a course comprised mostly, and at times, solely, of direct care workers, there may be a mistrust of management, instructors, and session content. Having previous positive relationships with some staff provided some credibility for me, and both instructors spent a considerable amount of time on the units getting to know staff. Roth and Calle-Mesa noted that the instructor's ability to convey a "genuine personal connection" (2006, p. 280) is key, especially when the instructor is of a different ethnicity and/or social class. In addition to a regular mindfulness practice, training and experience in teaching, instructors for courses with similar populations should be prepared for initial resistance or skepticism. An awareness of perceived differences and participants' rationale for these feelings is helpful. An instructor who consistently demonstrates sensitivity, authenticity, and compassion may well overcome initial reluctance, however.

Humor

Humor can provide connections when the instructor has a lighthearted approach. My co-teacher writes: "Humor can often be a universal language across cultural barriers. I remember when a lot of people got nervous around moving their body in the yoga class, giggling came up. Instead of trying to suppress it, allowing and celebrating the laughter sometimes helped—like playfully wiggling our hips to work out the kinks in our back" (Lombardo, personal communication, September 4, 2007).

Scheduling and Attendance

Nursing home and hospital staff can only be away from their responsibilities for brief periods, and staff "backfill," or replacements, are crucial to offering uninterrupted sessions with regular attendance. In addition, nursing homes are staffed 7 days a week, 24 hours a day. This means that scheduling a time when regular staff is consistently available is more difficult—staff schedules may change day to day, week to week. Evening and night sessions are also important. We found it helpful to work with nursing schedulers to maintain consistency. Despite our attempts, however, maintaining consistent staff members in these courses was a challenge.

Course attendance was irregular also. Sometimes, staff did not attend because they stated that the workload that met them when they returned to the unit destroyed any benefits they derived from the sessions. At times, I was discouraged by low attendance, but at other times, the impact of the course was apparent. One early morning I was walking to work as the night shift was leaving. The previous night, attendance was very low, and I wondered if this course was making a difference. I saw a group of nursing assistants gathered at a wall. One nursing assistant was showing the others a yoga stretch against the wall. When they saw me, they let me know that the exercises were helping them. In Chapter 12, I discuss alternative groups that may be more accessible for caregivers who would find it difficult to attend an ongoing course.

Focus on Short, Practical Skills

It doesn't take long to do it—just a few minutes, but it makes such a big difference.

When introducing stress reduction practices to an overwhelmed staff, we often focused on short practices, including those that could be done while waiting for a bus or in other moments of downtime. When brief meditations were introduced in MBEC sessions, participants would comment on how changed they felt afterward. By noting that this experience did not take long, we could discuss times during the day when they could take a meditation break.

Empowerment

If I put my mind on something to get it done, I will achieve my goal.

In mindfulness practice, letting go of goals and expectations is a fundamental tenet. When working with significantly disempowered populations, however, group outcomes may include improved self-esteem and a sense of internal control (Roth & Calle-Mesa, 2006, p. 266). Mindfulness connects practitioners with their own inner wisdom. Empowerment relocates control from external sources to internal resources. In this group, many caregivers of frail elders reported these benefits.

Shifts in Perception

I'm finding I'm more tense than I thought I was.
I like to enjoy my coffee in the a.m. when I am mindful eating [sic].

Class members consistently reported increased self-awareness. Discussion in class often focused on stressful situations at work and at home. The members found many of the skills learned in class helpful. Participants were able to share difficult work situations and strategize use of skills. There was a climate of nonjudgmental acceptance, allowing the group members to share their frustrations and feel connected and supported.

[I am learning] how to respond to stressful situations. [I am] able to react better when stressful situations occur. [I am] preparing myself that I become more stressed if I let everything—even simple things—stress me out.

Conclusion

> I remember thinking many times during the class that this work has a way of bringing us all to a common denominator. We all have bodies, breath, and thoughts. Many times I looked around thinking how cool it was that we were all from such different backgrounds, but could join together in this special way (A. Lombardo, personal communication, September 4, 2007).

A 7-week, 1-hour course for staff caregivers can offer significant benefits. Inclusion of night and evening shifts may be challenging for the instructors, but it is appreciated by these underserved caregivers. Direct caregivers may benefit from some adaptations and modifications. Roth and Calle-Mesa (2006) report that they did not utilize handouts, but did include a graduation with certificates. While we did not do either of these, I believe these adaptations are important to consider for this population. Also, when recruiting and introducing the class, the instructor's awareness of differing perceptions and expectations regarding classes is helpful.

Irregular attendance in this course was attributable to irregular work schedules and high work demands. Yet, staff anecdotal reports of this course's impact were overwhelmingly positive. I often found that when I visited the units, staff would come up to me and talk about something they had done mindfully. Staff also reported sharing the experiences in their home environment. One class member stated that she did not have time to practice on her own, but listened to the CD with her child at night. This class was held 5 years ago, and recently, I saw one of the participants. She told me she still plays the CD and practices what we learned together.

> I hope it will always continue. . . . Need this more often. . . . Keep classes on continuing basis. . . . Continue this next year. . . . More yoga! I really appreciate this class; I look forward to it.

REFERENCES

Nhat Hanh, T. (2001). *Anger: Wisdom for cooling the flames.* New York: Riverhead.
Roth, B., & Calle-Mesa, L. (2006). Mindfulness-Based Stress Reduction (MBSR) with Spanish- and English-speaking inner-city medical patients. In R. A. Baer (Ed.), *Mindfulness-based treatment approaches* (pp. 263–284). Burlington, MA: Elsevier.

CHAPTER 12

Introduction to Stress Reduction for Professional Caregivers: A 1-Hour Class and Other Options for Staff

---

DID I DO SOMETHING WRONG? (ED'S STORY)

Ed is a confused, pleasant, and mildly agitated nursing home resident. A chair alarm is attached to his sweater because he is at risk for falling out of his wheelchair. He cannot stand without assistance, and yet, he repeatedly tries to get up or to bend over to pick up something on the floor. The alarm is frequently set off and emits a loud beeping sound. Staff rush to replace Ed in the chair and to reinsert the alarm. The unit can be very busy and rescuing Ed many times is wearing. Staff may respond with increasing irritation or ask Ed to please stop bending down. Once, when I went to adjust the alarm, Ed looked up with the sweetest eyes and said, "Did I do something wrong?" Of course he did not, but the response of a stressed-out staff had caused him to think that he did.

Working with elders who are confused or who have significant care needs can be challenging. Most staff who choose this work say they want to help, they love older people, they feel a calling. And yet, caregiving can be stressful, impacting both the caregiver and the care receiver. Even without an ongoing, close relationship, stress is contagious on nursing home units. As discussed in Chapter 11, releasing staff for a 7-week, 1-hour course away from the nursing unit is beneficial. It is not always possible to release staff, however. This chapter offers alternative ways to introduce stress management and mindfulness to professional caregivers.

Mindfulness practices as traditionally taught require discipline and commitment. The programs and presentations described below do not require this commitment. Nevertheless, brief stress reduction programs introduce practices that can offer tools and strategies benefiting both caregivers and care receivers. For some participants, these presentations open the door to new practices and ways of perceiving.

PROFESSIONAL CAREGIVING

Demands of Elder Care

Residents and clients experience multiple losses, including their health, their friends and family, their homes, their roles in life, their ability to communicate, and their memory. At times, residents may feel sad, confused, or angry and project these feelings onto the care provider.

In the nursing home and community settings, demands on staff are often high. The most challenging care can be for those residents, like Ed, who are confused and agitated, putting themselves and others at risk if not closely supervised. Direct care staff may be providing care for one resident when another resident needs immediate assistance. Staff may have to make difficult choices during their entire shift. Persons in need of care may also be anxious and need constant reassurance. At times, staff may feel able to provide reassurance; at other times, they may feel hurried and pulled in many directions, unable to provide this support and reassurance.

Providing care for frail and dependent elders in an institutional or agency setting includes the additional responsibility of compliance to regulatory and agency standards, usually including extensive paperwork. In some situations, direct care staff feel they have little control over the day-to-day operations of the institution or agency. Culture Change models of care shift this paradigm, giving daily decision-making authority to those who will be implementing the decisions. (See Chapter 1 for Culture Change description.)

End-of-Life Care

Providing care for elders also often means providing end-of-life care. Most health care professionals have been trained to support and extend life. Providing comfort or end-of-life care can be difficult when direct care providers have personal relationships with the dying elder or due to religious and ethical concerns. Support for professional caregivers with ethical concerns or grief is often not built into institutional systems.

Families

Caregivers also interact with families and other informal caregivers. Care receivers and their families may have difficulty showing gratitude for the work done by care providers. Families may feel displaced and want to correct or instruct them. Nursing homes, in particular, receive press coverage for poor care, but not for the excellent daily care they provide. Professional caregivers may feel criticized or second-guessed by the informal caregivers, and hostile relations may escalate.

Results of High Stress in the Workplace

What happens when caregivers are overstressed at work? If they feel powerless to change their job stressors, they may respond in ways that include lackluster job performance, absenteeism, unwillingness to pitch in, negative behavior, or verbal comments that make residents and families feel fearful or jeopardized. Teamwork and camaraderie may decline on the units; staff may even sabotage each other or management. Injuries or accidents may increase and mistrust may develop. Use of alcohol and substance abuse may increase.

A 1-HOUR STRESS REDUCTION PROGRAM

One way to introduce the concepts of the mind-body connection and self-care for staff is a 1-hour presentation. The following describes a stress reduction class I offered at a large urban nursing home in collaboration with the Director of Psychiatry. For those staff already practicing some forms of self-care, it provided increased options. You may wish to use some or all of the information, tailoring the presentation to your needs and those of your institution, program, or agency.

Initial Considerations

The 1-hour presentation was open to all staff caregivers. Department heads were included in the planning of the schedule and encouraged to send their staff. Some departments made the presentation mandatory, and others did not. Group size ranged from 10–30 participants per session, and the majority of employees attended. Presentations were also scheduled for evening and night shifts and were held in a central area of the nursing home at multiple hours and days. Information on stress and a brief experiential session were included. Participants were given handouts with referrals to books, CDs, and other appropriate programs as well as some short mindfulness exercises to practice. (Some of the exercises are included in Appendices A, B, and D. Sample handouts are included in Appendix E.

The stress reduction presentation was promoted via departmental communications and postings throughout the nursing home using the words *stress management* or *stress reduction* because everyone seemed to identify with them!

Introduction

Stress is commonly acknowledged by staff, but the mind-body connection may not be clear to all. Therefore, it can be helpful to begin the presentation by asking staff to describe a particularly stressful incident at work. If participants are reluctant, offer some examples: the angry family walking in or the combative resident who needs to be bathed. Once participants identify a few situations, ask them if they can remember how they felt physically when the incident happened and where in their bodies they felt it. Staff generally respond well when examples that relate to their own experiences are used. Participants usually are able to identify where they felt the stress, with most identifying the stomach or shoulders or chest. If the group is quiet at this point, I use myself as an example, sharing where I physically experienced stress. This concrete, personal example was one useful way to establish the connection between the mind and the body. Following this introduction, the class was divided into two segments: a presentation on the causes, effects, and strategies for coping with stress; and an experiential section that included stretches, breathing exercises, and a brief guided meditation.

Psychoeducational Presentation on Stress Management

The educational component of the class defined stress—what it is, and its effect on us. Caregivers are often very interested in this subject because of the personal impact. I used a PowerPoint presentation, which I made interactive, engaging the group with examples from their daily lives. The following section details the information I presented on stress and the mind–body connection, general coping strategies, and specific ones for dealing with the stresses of caregiving for frail elders. It is also helpful to include the specific stressors of caregiving in the nursing home, normalizing many aspects of this challenging care.

STAFF PSYCHOEDUCATIONAL PRESENTATION ON STRESS

Below are highlights of this presentation, illustrated with examples relevant to nursing home employees (adapted in part from Lantz, 2000).

What Is Stress?

Stress Links Our Mind and Our Body

Stress has physical symptoms that were appropriate for cave dwellers, but not necessarily for humans in the 21st century. When we are very stressed, our body goes into high alert: fight or flight. For our predecessors, these reactions were life-prolonging. Stressors that people cope with today are quite different, and fight or flight is no longer appropriate. Consider the common situation of a resident who does not want to eat despite encouragement and assistance. The resident's family has complained of neglect to the nursing home administrator. It is not a situation where it would be helpful for a caregiver to run away or start a fight. If the caregiver's body is responding to the stress, however, and this stress is unresolved and prolonged, chronic stress and the accompanying physical symptoms may arise.

What Is Stressful to Me Is Not Necessarily Stressful to You

Why does the same external event that stresses me out cause you to smile and shrug your shoulders? Consider flying or public speaking. For some, these are traumatic experiences. Other people enjoy, or, at least, don't mind them. *Whatever life offers us, the events are perceived uniquely by each of us.* Conveying this concept is crucial to understanding and engaging our response to stress. It also implies that we take responsibility for our reaction to stress rather than solely blaming the external event.

Stress Can Feel Overwhelming

Two basic causes of stress are high expectations and low control. When we are not clear about what is expected of us, or we feel unsupported, we become stressed. We not only can feel anxious, but if stressed for a long period of time, we may become depressed. The emotional strain can lead to social isolation, guilt, anger, frustration, and resentment. Stress is a part of life, but overwhelming chronic stress has long- and short-term impact on our health and functioning.

What Can We Do About Stress?

Healthy Stress

Stress is also associated with that which we aspire to and value. Going back to school, raising a family, and seeking a promotion are all stressful, and also, are rewarding. Stress, in itself, is not bad. Chronic unresolved stress may lead to physical and psychological distress, inadequate job performance, and unhealthy coping. Healthy stress, however, can lead to growth and development. We can achieve our highest goals when we challenge ourselves and take risks and opportunities.

The Role of Perception and Stress

If stress is related to how we perceive our lives, a crucial element in stress reduction is to consider how we interpret what happens to us. Consider the resident who does not want to be washed. The resident might even be physically or verbally abusive. Caregivers may feel angry with the resident because he is making the job more difficult and is not appreciative of the care we provide. Caregivers might feel nervous because they may be held responsible if the resident looks disheveled or dirty. Or, caregivers might feel compassion for the resident who could be confused and frightened. Any of these interpretations result in different feelings. Consider how the interpretations of this event could lead to different emotions and responses.

Observe Helpful and Unhelpful Thoughts

An important first step in reducing stress is taking a moment to step back and consider how you perceive events. Unhelpful thoughts can include assigning blame to others for our feelings: "You make me so angry"; generalized negative thinking: "Nobody cares here"; and wishing things could be different than they are: "If only I could win the lottery." Research on cognitive therapy has shown that negative thoughts often lead to depression. When we learn to observe our thoughts and make choices, we can choose to accept responsibility for our feelings, view the world in a more balanced way, and accept where we are in any given moment. We might even say helpful thoughts to ourselves such as: "I am proud of the work I do"; "There are residents and families who really appreciate me"; "I like myself." Learning to accept our limits can empower us more than striving for an impossible perfection.

Understanding Our Own Stressors

We are the experts in our own stress—what causes us tension, worry, and anxiety, and what helps. Becoming familiar with our own symptoms of stress can give early warning signs so that we can take care of ourselves rather than let stress build up. Learning to pay more attention to our body's signals is a first step.

Making Helpful Choices

Even in the most challenging of work environments, we have control of how we respond. Caregivers have some choices, like the extra few minutes spent taking care of the resident's hair or discussing her granddaughter's graduation. In situations where staff feel unsupported, encourage them to congratulate themselves and each other for the good work they do.

Caregiving Rewards

Caregiving for older adults clearly has rewards. Professional caregivers are proud of the services they provide. Even when they feel close to burnout and desperately need these classes, they know they are doing valuable work. They have expertise and personal knowledge in an important field. They often form intimate relationships with those for whom they provide care and with their families. Elders and their families are frequently very grateful for their caring services.

Most staff know that they make a difference and that small kindnesses matter. Everyone can be a positive force in the work environment. Stress is contagious, but a calm and compassionate presence is also contagious. Become involved in changes in the workplace that help.

Stress Busters and Lifestyle Changes

There are strategies for responding to stressful circumstances as they arise, such as taking a time-out or a few moments to deep breathe and stretch. Also, consider lifestyle changes that reduce stress in the long run such as regular exercise programs, meditation, diet, and mindfulness.

EXPERIENTIAL EXERCISES

Following the psychoeducational presentation on stress, participants can be invited to discuss what they already do to help with job and personal stress.

I may remind them of the earlier question about where they feel tension in their bodies. This can also serve to introduce the experiential portion of the program in which participants practice yoga, deep breathing, and a guided body scan. It is most helpful for caregiving staff to begin to understand stress from their own personal experiences—in their own minds and bodies. It is the motivator for change.

These experiences provided participants a way to learn from the inside out about the mind–body connection. Appendix A describes simple standing, and chair, yoga stretches appropriate for those in work clothing and without any yoga experience. Below, I highlight some suggestions for instructors.

Yoga Poses

- It is important to remind participants to pay attention to their bodies, following only instructions that feel right for them.
- Demonstrate by doing the pose yourself. Observe the group members during the poses.
- Offer encouragement and verbal adjustments. At the same time, participants may be self-conscious, so keep a lighthearted attitude.

Deep Breathing

- Practice the deep breathing with the group, demonstrating by having them put their hands on their belly, then ribs, then upper chest.
- Encourage participants to breathe very slowly and deeply.
- When they finish, ask them to note how they are feeling.
- Point out that deep breathing is one way to use our breath, different from awareness of breathing.
- Emphasize that it is something they can use for on-the-spot stress reduction.

Guided Meditation and/or a Body Scan

- A shortened breath awareness or a body scan can be adapted from the script in Appendix B.
- Practice this experience yourself before guiding others. CDs are available with guided meditations and body scans.
- The scripts are only for guidance and should not be read.
- At the end, try a few more simple chair stretches with the group.

Appendix B provides scripts for breathing exercises, body scan, guided meditation, and a reference guide for more resources. Instructors should be personally familiar with the exercises they choose to use. Before teaching yoga and meditation, study with a professional yoga instructor and have a regular yoga and meditation practice. It is important that instructors personalize the presentation of the exercises, so that they sound and feel individualized, not formatted. A composed and authentic instructor conveys compassion, acceptance, and humor.

Conclusion of the Presentation

- End the group by asking group members to note how they are feeling in their bodies.
- Conclude with a discussion on incorporating stress management and mindfulness into the very real, very busy lives that we all have.
- Ask staff to identify some stressful work situations and strategize ways of de-stressing, so that the situation can be responded to more skillfully. Emphasize that most of what we practiced in class is available to them at any time. Many of the practices can be done while waiting for a bus or in the car at a traffic light. Some of the quick stretches can be done during a short break.
- Sample handouts, available in Appendix E, can reinforce practical ways to integrate simple, short practices into a daily routine.

Most important, reinforce that caregiving work can be stressful and encourage staff to care for themselves as well as they care for our residents and their families.

- Initially, it is most helpful and realistic to integrate small changes into our lives. Regular practice is also essential.
- As with any skill, the more we use it, the more we are likely to use it again. If we take deep breaths in the shower every morning, or sit in meditation at the beginning of our day, we may find ourselves handling stressful situations differently.

The 1-hour stress class introduces many important concepts. You may be asked to make referrals. It can be helpful to have information available on local programs, Internet sites, and a reading list. (See Appendix F for referrals.) During these sessions, you may identify some staff in personal crisis or with serious, unresolved issues. In your presentation, communicate that simply talking about a problem can make us feel better. Suggest staff talk to a friend or to a religious or counseling professional when needed. You may also want to have a list of local counseling agencies or other referrals available.

Participant Response

Simple feedback forms and spontaneous verbal responses were overwhelmingly positive. During our feedback discussion, participants verbalized what they had experienced during the groups. Some said they felt more relaxed. Some said they found a quiet place inside. Some said they felt physically better. Many expressed an interest in follow-up classes.

ALTERNATE OPTIONS FOR SHORT STRESS REDUCTION SESSIONS

A 1-hour stress reduction program away from the work environment may be effective in introducing stress reduction and mindfulness to staff, but not all staff will be reached in this way. Many find it hard to leave their work, aside from brief meal breaks. Their workload may be difficult to complete, and they may not feel they have the time. Others may be reluctant to participate in these novel groups and experiences.

An option to consider is running stress reduction classes on the nursing home units. While most nursing home units are not conducive to stress reduction, it is the place where staff spend most of their time. Learning to feel less stressed there may demonstrate to staff that it is possible to reduce stress and even meditate in a noisy, busy environment. The remainder of this chapter reviews three options to consider.

Mini Stress Reduction Sessions on the Nursing Units

A series of short (15–30 minutes) stress reduction sessions can be adapted for staff on the nursing units or other work environments. It is helpful to talk with them about timing; there is a rhythm to their day, and some times are better than others for a break. Some may come in to the session on time, and others may come in 5, 10, or even 15 minutes late. It is important to allow staff to partake in whatever way they can and not to make an issue of lateness. The sessions can have a theme like healthy eating, or chronic pain, or aromatherapy. In general, sessions include stretches and meditation, discussion and experience. (See Appendix D for some ideas for brief sessions.)

Residents and Staff Together: A Model for Culture Change

Initial MBEC groups were for residents on the nursing home units, usually in the dining area. Staff began to bring their paperwork into that room. They sat at the opposite end of the room, but were clearly there to participate in the calming environment of aromatherapy, music, and relaxation exercises. Some staff members even stated that they looked forward to the weekly group or asked me where to buy the essential oils for aromatherapy or the stress management CDs. I began to ask staff to join us. From then on, two or three nursing assistants would participate, sitting in meditation, doing the stretches, and sharing in the discussion. This group of residents and staff together was very powerful.

As the nursing home transitioned to a Culture Change Community, these resident/caregiver groups served as models for a shared community. While previous groups did not exclude staff and other caregivers, these groups were designed to encourage a broader membership. Sessions were scheduled on both day and evening shifts, and we also invited informal caregivers. Private paid companions regularly joined us, and at times, families. Participating in mindfulness groups together provides skills, tools, and understanding that empower direct care staff and residents to develop a relationship with their own strengths and knowledge base.

A Wellness Coordinator

Following the 7-week class for staff reported in Chapter 11, the units who participated had 100% staff retention. In addition, staff satisfaction surveys demonstrated improvement in nursing satisfaction. Although there may have been other factors involved, the benefits of the program were apparent, and a Wellness Coordinator was hired for staff.

The Wellness Coordinator was responsible for regular programs for all three sites of this large urban nursing home with nearly 1,800 employees. Employees comprised a large variety of ethnicities and cultures. Programs were offered on all three shifts, including evening and night. In addition, individual work could be scheduled as requested and indicated. The Wellness Coordinator was also the instructor for the 7-week class and a research study discussed in Section IV. She was known to staff, accepted, and well versed in a large range of health topics. As discussed in detail in Chapter 11, the *presence* of the instructor is essential when approaching a large mixed audience that may include persons from a variety of ethnicities and socio-economic status.

The first step was to administer a needs assessment for staff. An inclusive questionnaire was distributed with their paychecks (a great way to get attention!). This Wellness Survey provided an introduction to the program and set a friendly nonjudgmental tone. Responders were told there were no right and wrong answers, responses were anonymous, and completion was voluntary, as was skipping questions. The one-page (two-sided) survey assessed current information on physical activity, nutrition, and program interests. Aside from introducing the program and gathering information, it was hoped that staff would feel that their input was an important part of the program. An initial assessment also established a baseline for staff health behaviors in these areas. In addition to the written survey, we met with small focus groups of staff and department heads.

Once the results of the survey were tabulated, the Wellness Coordinator designed a simple format: one wellness theme each month was presented in 1-hour sessions. Wellness themes included mindfulness, breathing exercises, healthy eating, aromatherapy, meditation, mood management, yoga, self-massage, guided imagery, and managing chronic pain. These topics were presented at a variety of times in an experiential manner (A. Lombardo, personal communication, August 30, 2007). The programs were for staff benefit. For participants unfamiliar with the previous 7-week class, it was important to establish a trusting supportive environment. Handouts were provided and home practice was encouraged. A brief survey was given out at the end of each class for feedback.

Response to this program was overwhelmingly positive: 98% of attendees said they would like more training in related subjects. Total attendance for the 1-year program was 1,772 staff visits. Consistent attendance continued to be problematic, however. Programs such as this, while effective, would benefit from increased coordination with other programs and integration into the home's infrastructure.

COMMENTS FROM STAFF

Finally! An in-service I can use at home!
This is excellent in the overwhelming job we have.
This is the best part of my week. This should be required.
It is very good that the Home thinks about their employees' well-being.
This was helpful for many of my pains.
I feel so good!
We need more of this! Please give us more training on this.
Please continue to have sessions. I am learning much and sharing it with others.

CONCLUSION

The brief stress reduction programs for staff in health care settings are one way to introduce the concepts and practices of mindfulness, meditation, and yoga to an audience that might not otherwise have encountered them. Based on these short classes, many of the staff reported continued use of the skills at work and in their personal lives. This chapter intends to provide a good starting point for similar programs. For specific exercises and handouts, see Appendices D and E.

In addition to presenting this information, you can teach these strategies by embodying them!

RECOMMENDATIONS

Dedicated staff, space, and resources are essential to fully integrating wellness into a health care facility. Nevertheless, smaller programs have impacted staff and residents in many powerful ways. Moving forward to a Culture Change philosophy, classes that include staff, residents, and informal caregivers could promote collaboration and connection. Management participation at all levels also sends an important message and could help managers with their own stress. In addition to offering classes, facilities could consider a mindfulness corner, or bulletin board, with quotes for the day or the week. Staff could choose mindfulness buddies to check in with when they are feeling stressed. Aromatherapy is also a great quick connection for staff. We often carry around perfume sticks with essential oils on them. Staff are always amazed at how something as simple as a certain scent can shift their mood (A. Lombardo, personal communication, August 30, 2007).

REFERENCE

Lantz, M. S. (2000). Staff presentation, Jewish Home and Hospital, New York.

SECTION IV

Conclusions

CHAPTER 13

Walking With Tigers

Aging is not what happens to someone else. It is happening to us, moment by moment. It is us, but older.

A STORY

Ajahn Mun, a Thai monk of the forest tradition, chose to live in an area that was teeming with wild tigers. He and his monks practiced mindful walking outside, sometimes at night. Occasionally, the tigers were close by and could be heard growling. At times, they did not harm the monks. At other times, they did. The monks found that this practice provided a sense of the immediacy and importance to each moment. And we all live with tigers of some sort. (Liebenson Grady, 1996)

Elders and their caregivers may feel as though they are walking with tigers, too. Many elders have discovered through loss and suffering what mindfulness practice teaches—everything changes. We will grow old, we will become ill, we will lose all that is precious and dear to us, we will die.

DEFINING AGING

This book has cited many difficulties that elders face, but the elders are not the problem. The limitations lie in the institutions and services (or lack of them) and in our individual and corporate denial of aging. Over 30 years ago, Barry Barkan began advocating for elders, seeing them as a disempowered minority and their treatment as a civil rights issue.

DEFINITION OF AN ELDER

An Elder is a person who is still growing, still a learner, still with potential, and whose life continues to have within it, promise for and connection to the future. An Elder is still in pursuit of happiness, joy and pleasure, and her or his birthright to these remains intact. Moreover, an Elder is a person who deserves respect and honor and whose work is to synthesize wisdom from long life experience and formulate this into a legacy for future generations.

Barry Barkan, Live Oak Institute, 1976

Aging Successfully, Conscious Aging, and Sage-ing

H. R. Moody (2003) differentiates "successful aging" from "conscious aging." Both models offer benefits and are not necessarily mutually exclusive. In successful aging, change is adaptive, modifying the impact of aging on appearance and health. Similar to conventional medical systems that seek to defeat illness, those who desire to age successfully may also endeavor to defeat aging. This model carries important benefits. It dispels the perception of aging as a time solely of deterioration and decline. It provides evidence-based strategies for enhancing quantity and quality of life for elders.

Conscious aging is holistic and transformational. Change is internal and fundamental. Conscious aging may be more challenging in that it asks the individual to take responsibility for deep, genuine, personal investigation. When we age consciously, we do not endeavor to defeat, defy, or deny aging; we seek to accept, learn, and grow from it. Many have found this model to be helpful in situations that cannot be changed or cured.

One path to conscious aging, called Spiritual Eldering, or Sage-ing, a program introduced by Rabbi Schachter-Shalomi in *From Age-ing to Sage-ing* (1995), has been taken by elders working together in groups. These groups practice meditation, forgiveness, journaling and drawing, and guided imagery to deepen their understanding of their own aging and spiritual path. Schachter-Shalomi defined elders as potential sages:

> Sages draw on growth techniques from modern psychology and contemplative practices from the world's spiritual traditions to expand their consciousness and develop wisdom. By expressing this wisdom as consecrated service to the community, they endow their lives with meaning and avoid becoming economic and psychological burdens on their loved ones and on society. This ongoing process, which I call *spiritual eldering*, helps us consciously transform the downward arc of aging into the upward arc of

expanded consciousness that crowns an elder's life with meaning and purpose. (Schachter-Shalomi, 1995, pp. 5–6)

Conventional health care institutions generally offer a specialized, hierarchical, pathology-based model. These models have brought relief and cure to countless individuals and their families. CAM, Culture Change, and other such models offer a palliative, quality-of-life, patient- and resident-focused, holistic, and strength-based approach to care. CAM and Culture Change require transformational, not incremental, change. These models have engendered growth and provided comfort for many. Fortunately, health care consumers do not have to choose. Used individually, with discretion or in consort, these models increase our healing options. Both serve those who need care and those who give care.

CARING FOR ELDERS, CARING FOR OURSELVES

Mindfulness-Based Elder Care promotes interventions and programs designed to engage frail elders and their caregivers in the process of conscious aging. These programs and courses take place for the most part in the context of the current nursing home environment. While MBEC and other add-on programs may offer relief, another approach is to transform the institutional structure itself. Below are three models of institutional innovation and my own vision.

The Zen Hospice

The Zen Hospice in San Francisco was the first hospice organization grounded in mindfulness. Founding Director Frank Ostaseski describes the underlying philosophy as mutual service.

> I think it's helpful to start with the basic, but true premise that real service does not happen unless both people are being served. . . . I do this work because I love it and because it serves me. I try to see myself in each person that I serve, and I try to see them in me. . . . You see, at the very heart of service we understand that the act of caring is always mutually beneficial. We understand that in nurturing others we are always caring for ourselves, and this understanding fundamentally shifts the way we provide care. (Ostaseski, 1996).

Caregivers at the Zen Hospice bring mindfulness and compassion to their care of the dying. By focusing on connections and presence, caregivers experience the mutuality of the relationship and are less likely to get burnt out.

Being with death and dying can bring increased awareness of our own mortality. It can be uncomfortable or distressing. It can also lead to increased comfort with life's transience and increased enjoyment of each moment.

The Eden Alternative or the Green House Model

Bill Thomas calls nursing homes a "relic" and compares their "institutional" model of care to prisons (Thomas, 2002). He goes on to say that the solution is multifaceted; there should be "a thousand flavors." Thomas's model, a Green House, for care of frail elders is small, warm, and resident-centered. In addition, he integrates plants, animals, and children into his Green Houses. Thomas puts *Shahbazim*, nursing assistants, in a leadership role, empowering those who are closest to the elder. Shahbazim are responsible for sustaining the elder in body and spirit. Relationships are central, and nurture both caregiver and care receiver. At the core of the Eden Alternative philosophy is the desire to "do good deeds without expectation of any return" (Thomas, 2004, p. 210). Thomas also cites the importance of "being" as well as "doing," defining childhood and elderhood as a time of being and middle age as a time of doing (p. 118).

L'Arche

In 1964, Jean Vanier, moved by compassion and a desire to "do good," and brought three previously institutionalized men with mental disabilities to live with him. This first community was in France and came to be known as l'Arche. There are now 120 similar models in 30 different countries. The values and beliefs of l'Arche are reflected in its name, which translates as "the ark," a vessel that represents all of creation, traveling together. Caregivers are "assistants" and care receivers are "core members." They live together in small homes where relationships are the priority and viewed as enhancing the lives of all. Assistants at l'Arche focus on commonalities with those they care for, rather than differences. They recognize that they learn about joy, presence, and courage from the core members. Vanier states: "We all have to reflect on how we're in front of pain. We're all running away from it, we can't stand it, we don't know what to do with it. We don't know what to do with the beggar crying out. We find all sorts of reasons not to look at him. And the whole question is how to stand before pain" (American Public Radio, 2007).

These three models care for different populations, and yet share a similar philosophy and approach to care. They value relationship and view the bonds between those who need care and those who give care as mutually growth promoting and enhancing. Relationships are not between helper and helped, professional and patient, but acknowledge the fullness and wounds we all carry. These models focus on the person, not the disability. They describe a small, healing, nurturing environment. They recognize that the basic needs to connect with others and to feel valued and accepted are common to all humanity. Compassion and presence are central.

True Home for Elders

Your true home is in the here and the now. It is not limited by time, space, nationality, or race. Your true home is not an abstract idea. It is something you can touch and live in every moment. (Nhat Hanh, 2006)

Consider this idea: "True Home for Elders": elder care provided in small homes, grounded in (nondenominational) mindfulness practice. Rather than as add-on programs, in these homes, the mindfulness principles of relationship, compassion, and presence are core.

Our philosophy of care is often reflected in the way we describe those who need care, those who give care, and the places and ways care is given. Bill Thomas has used Green House and Eden Alternative to convey the importance of place and even created a new word with Persian and Hebrew roots—*Shahbazim*—to identify caregivers in his model (2004, p. 254). At l'Arche, care models are called "communities"; care receivers, "core members"; and care providers, "assistants."

True Home for Elders will provide mindfulness-based residential care for elders who need supervision but not necessarily extensive nursing care. Elders with dementia can be the most challenging to care for at home due to their increasingly unsafe behaviors. Traditional nursing homes care for all elders in a similar medically modeled manner that often contradicts the needs of those with dementia. True Home's approach will be supportive rather than restrictive, reducing the potential for behavioral problems. Mindful interventions may also take advantage of the knowledge of both Western and Eastern traditions of healing. While True Home for Elders will promote conscious aging, medical treatment and intervention will be utilized and integrated as needed and desired by elders and their families.

The communities also will offer opportunities for volunteers to serve and to experience mindful presence in action. One practice employed in MBSR training is an aikido exercise. Participants act out varied ways of responding to undesired events, embodied by another participant rushing at them. Response choices include passivity (lying down); avoidance (stepping aside); aggression (physically confronting). The aikido alternative engages the aggressor, embracing or holding hands while moving together. Connecting with frail elders means engaging with our own tigers: perhaps fear of illness, death, or loss; perhaps our reactions to agitated and aggressive behaviors. At True Home for Elders, volunteers will be encouraged to practice mindfulness with compassion and insight, in relationship with each other and with elders, possibly confused and agitated elders. Resembling the Zen Hospice, True Home for Elders, though founded in mindfulness practice, will not be limited to practitioners. It will be open to any volunteer who views service as integral to a spiritual path. Volunteers who are not mindfulness practitioners can be trained in mindfulness practices.

Formal programs of mindfulness meditation and yoga will also be offered in this setting for both elders and caregivers. As this book describes, confused elders respond well to MBEC practices. With mindful practice at the home's core, caregivers will engage those they care for in ways that decrease rather than increase distress.

True Home for Elders will place elders and those closest to them at the center of decision making, reflecting the Eden Alternative and other Culture Change communities. Treatment modalities will include CAM, nature, animals, children, and creativity. Similar to l'Arche, caregiving staff will be empowered and encouraged to engage with elders on an individual basis, making connections and forming relationships.

The need for change in long-term care as well as the barriers to change have been well documented by the Pioneer Network, the Paraprofessional Healthcare Institute, and Thomas. There are clearly obstacles to implementing True Homes for Elders. Agencies and homes that provide elder care are highly regulated. These regulations were enacted to protect elders, and yet, have yielded a system that frequently values compliance and paperwork over relationships. Currently, enlightened regulators are engaging professionals who desire change. It is hoped increased flexibility will transpire in the future. Reimbursement systems also need examination. There are some excellent assisted living facilities modeled on CAM, but they are only available to individuals who can pay privately. There are other questions that will need to be resolved: What happens when elders need more care? How would it be paid for? How would regulations be complied with? "Making the dream come true—that is the thing. . . . The reality is, of course, more complicated than the dream" (Thomas, 2004, p. 209). The three models above demonstrate dreams can become a reality.

Let us end as we began, by observing the evolution of health care. "Culture and norms are not static; they are always in transition. Usually, we envision the way things are as the way they should be. It is hard to imagine things being different. Fortunately, when we realize that some alteration must happen and that the old way of functioning is limited, the need to change surpasses the challenges inherent in the change process."

IMAGINE THIS

You can no longer function independently. You need to leave the home you have lived in and move to a communal setting. What would you want in place? What would make this move acceptable to you? Would you want pets, if you have them? A kitchen? Your own room?

Elders are not different, they are just us, but older.

FOR YOU

This book emphasizes the importance of the instructor's presence, but presence is a tiger, it requires clear and compassionate honesty. It takes commitment and energy not to fall back on routine behaviors and roles, to understand what is called for in each unique interaction. Caregivers engaged with the models of Zen Hospice, Green House, and l'Arche find strength in their relationships with elders, core members, and dying patients. The authentic presence they bring to these relationships nurtures both.

The first step is often the most daunting to novice practitioners and teachers. MBEC programs began with small, mindfulness meditation groups in a nursing home. Over time, they had a significant impact on the institution. The most profound changes, often, are from the bottom up.

So, this book is for you: the elders, the professional caregivers, and the families and friends who continue to care for their elders, whether at home or in a long-term-care setting. Systemic change is occurring, expanding the vision to include both curing and caring. It is important to ensure that change is fundamental and not superficial. There is room for many approaches to care. You can be a part of this change. What is your vision?

REFERENCES

American Public Radio. (2007, August 2). *L'Arche, a community of brokenness and beauty.* Retrieved August 2, 2007, from http://speakingoffaith.publicradio.org/programs/larche/transcript.shtml

Liebenson Grady, M., & Liebenson Grady, N. (1996, Fall). Investigation: Listening as deeply as we possibly can. *Insight, 7,* 36–39. Article excerpted from a program offered at the Barre Center for Buddhist Studies on October 21, 1995.

Moody, H. R. (2003). Conscious Aging: A strategy for positive change in later life. In J. Ronch & J. Goldfield (Eds.), *Mental wellness in aging: Strength-based approaches* (pp. 139–160). Baltimore, MD: Human Professionals Press.

Nhat Hanh, T. (2006). Returning home. *Shambhala Sun, 33,* 58–63.

Ostaseski, F. (1996, November). *Zen Hospice project . . . Being of service.* Retrieved September 19, 2007, from http://urbandharma.org/udharma3/service.html

Schachter-Shalomi, Z., & Miller, R. (1995). *From Age-ing to Sage-ing: A profound new vision of growing older.* New York: Warner.

Thomas, W. H. (2002, October). *& Thou Shalt Honor.* Retrieved September 10, 2007, from http://www.pbs.org/thoushalthonor/eden/index.html

Thomas, W. H. (2004). *What are old people for? How elders will save the world.* Acton, MA: VanderWyk & Burnham.

SECTION V

Appendices

Mindfulness-Based Elder Care Yoga

OVERVIEW

The physical practice of yoga, called yoga asanas, teaches us to listen to our bodies. The yoga and mindfulness offered in this appendix are not about striving or reaching any particular pose and are especially helpful for elders and others whose bodies may not be agile or strong. This yoga is internal, working with our limits—both physical and emotional—attending to what is still available. Understanding the basic principles of yoga will help in considering adaptations for particular groups and settings.

STRETCHING

Yoga can teach us to listen to what feels right to us. It will be different from what feels right to our neighbors. Physical stretches can help us to become more limber and flexible. It allows us to explore our edges. It is also important not to push ourselves too far or too fast. Stretching too far can teach us about the consequences of not listening to what is right for us.

BALANCING

Balancing is not something you can think about doing, it only happens when you let go and let it happen. Or sometimes, it doesn't. When we lose our balance, how do we respond? Can we be compassionate with ourselves? We may even find that some days it is easier to maintain a balance than other days.

TRANSITIONS

I often tell people that Hatha Yoga is a practice in awareness, in paying attention to how we move into the pose, hold the pose and move out of the pose. That's why they are poses and not exercises: the awareness makes them poses allowing us to listen to our bodies (L. Sierra, personal communication, August 15, 2007).

As this experienced yoga teacher shares, paying attention to the entire practice is another way of being mindful. We may find that in the bigger picture of our lives, transition times are mindless. Transitions, whether big or small, can be times when we feel unengaged, unfocused. When we are experiencing big transitions in our life, we may desire to grasp onto an activity or goal. It can also be a time to practice being with what is, even if that is "not knowing."

LETTING GO

Yoga yokes the opposites of effort and ease. Effort gives us the strength to hold the pose, but we also need ease, a letting go. Yoga poses may remind us of this duality. Savasana, the corpse pose, gives us a chance to practice letting go. In this pose, we lie on our backs on the floor and release, allowing the floor to completely support us. This position may bring increased awareness regarding where we are holding tension in our bodies—and perhaps in our thoughts and emotions. We may find it takes "effort" to "let go." The balance of yoga, as often revealed in the corpse pose, is "effortless effort," or letting go of "trying."

FLEXING AND EXTENDING THE SPINE

It may be helpful to consider a series of movements, especially of the spine, and to adapt them to seated or prone positions. A twist, for example, can be done standing, seated, or prone. The cat and cow poses alternate arching the back forward and curving it backward. They also can be done, with modifications, lying down, seated, kneeling, or standing. Stretching upward with the arms and downward with the feet can be done in almost any position. Bending over can be done from a standing or a seated position.

Yoga allows us to discover our limits and also to experience our strengths and abilities. We also may find that our assumptions are erroneous—everything changes. For persons who may be focused on loss and disabilities, yoga offers more than stretches! Below are some suggested poses and adaptations. In working with yourself and others, yoga can be a time to focus inward with mindful awareness of physical sensations. If any pose does not feel comfortable, or you need to move, do so. Pay attention to your breath and move in harmony with it.

SUGGESTIONS FOR ELDERS IN WHEELCHAIRS

In each pose, remind elders to do only what feels right to them. Encourage participants to pay attention to body sensations and honor them. At the same time, encourage physical exploration and stretching in new ways. Demonstrate the poses yourself and also be prepared to offer hands-on assistance. Go slowly. Offer lots of encouragement and praise.

SUGGESTIONS FOR STAFF

Staff may be self-conscious about their bodies and lack of flexibility. For the instructor, it is helpful to be very supportive and also silly. Have fun. Let the atmosphere be playful. Staff will usually do chair and standing yoga.

STANDING STRETCHES

- Stand behind your chair, making sure there is enough space around to stretch in either direction.
- Take a few moments to become aware of standing. Notice any and all physical sensations.
- If comfortable, close your eyes, if not, find a spot on the floor to look at. The intention is to turn the focus inward.
- Reaching up, stretch all the way up to the ceiling. See if you can feel the stretch in all your joints.
- Don't forget to breathe!
- After stretching straight up, reach from side to side, stretching first one side, then the other.
- Now, stretch out and forward, if it is comfortable for you.
- Those with high blood pressure may not want to bend forward, but for the rest, reach out and over, coming slowly down toward the floor. Allow the body to stay in this inversion if it feels right to you, perhaps gently swinging from side to side, stretching in any way that feels good.

- When you feel ready, bend the knees and slowly straighten the back, coming up, vertebra by vertebra, until you are standing gently erect again.
- Close your eyes if it is comfortable to you, and notice how your body is feeling. Where do you feel your breath? What else do you notice?
- What would your life be like if sometimes you just stopped and took a moment to stand with awareness?

CHAIR YOGA

Shoulder Rolls

- Sitting up straight, inhale, and draw your shoulders up toward your ears.
- Now, roll your shoulders forward as if they could meet in front of you.
- Circle your shoulders down and then bring them back, feeling your shoulder blades draw together behind you.

Move slowly and breathe deeply, repeating three times or more. Then reverse the direction for three more circles.

Neck Rolls

- Sitting up straight, take a breath in, and without scrunching the back of the neck, look up toward the ceiling and look down.
- Roll the head from side to side as you look down.
- Come up and let the head drop to the right.
- If desired, take the right hand to the left ear to gently increase the stretch, only as far as is comfortable.
- Come back to center, and let the head drop to the left shoulder. You may notice that the shoulder hunches up toward the ear. If it does, relax the shoulder down.
- Again, the left hand can be placed on the right ear to intensify the stretch, if desired.
- Stretch only as far as is comfortable.

Leg and Ankle

- Sitting upright in the chair, lift your legs until they are straight in front of you, or as high as feels comfortable and safe.
- Flex your feet toward the ceiling, and point them straight out in front of you.

- Do this three times.
- Then, keep your legs raised and make circles with your feet and ankles, first in one direction, then the other.
- Lower your legs and see if you notice any physical sensations in your legs. You may notice a change, or not.

Arm and Wrist

- Bring your arms straight out in front of you and parallel.
- Flex and point your hands three times with the in and out breath.
- Then, slowly circle your hands in one direction and then the other, three times.
- When completed, shake your hands and arms as if you were shaking off water.
- Return your arms to your lap and note any sensations in your hands, wrists, arms, fingers, or shoulders.

Arms Overhead

- Inhale deeply as you raise your arms out to your sides and overhead, palms facing upward.
- Stretch up, feeling the stretch in your whole upper body—your fingers, wrists, arms, shoulders, ribs, and torso.
- Stretch up high on one side and then the other. Imagine there is something up high that you want, and reach for it! Don't forget to breathe.
- Slowly bring the arms down, moving as if through a thick liquid.
- When the arms come to rest, notice any sensations following this stretch—perhaps increased space in your joints or an increased awareness of the rib cage.

Side Stretch

- Stretch up overhead, or as high as you comfortably can, with arms parallel while making sure the shoulders feel open and broad.
- Now stretch over to one side.
- Come up and stretch to the other side.
- Do this two more times.
- Slowly, slowly, bring your arms down to your lap.

Back and Forward Bends

- Slowly raise the arms overhead or as high as is comfortable.
- Lift the arms slightly backward, opening the chest, and notice how you may be able to breathe in even more deeply.

- Slowly come forward, leading with the arms.
- Come as far forward as is beneficial for you—letting your hands go toward the floor. Your hands may reach the floor, your lap, or you may wish to rest your folded arms on your lap. Find a position of ease.
- When you are bent forward, stay there for a few breaths and notice where you feel your breath. This is intended to be a resting pose; so see if you can allow your body to release into it.
- After a few breaths, slowly uncurl the back, vertebra by vertebra, until you are in an upright position again.

Spinal Twists

- On an inhale, straighten up your spine in the chair.
- Slowly begin to twist around to the right, starting with your hips, then ribs.
- Place your left hand on your right knee or thigh.
- Twist your shoulders and place your right hand on the chair or arm of the chair. Finally, turn your neck and head to look behind you if that feels safe in your neck.
- See if you can stay in this position for three to five full breaths. With each in breath, lift up through the crown of your head, and with each out breath, twist a little more, if possible. Keep lengthening your spine.
- Slowly unwind the twist, and come back to center on the exhalation.
- Repeat for three to five breaths on the other side.

Eye Yoga

- Sitting, standing, or lying comfortably, begin by looking up with only your eyes. Don't move your head or neck.
- Now, look down with your eyes.
- Do this a few more times.
- Come back to center and slowly look side to side.
- Now, make a circle with your eyes, going very slowly in one direction three times and slowly in the other direction three times.
- Finish by closing your eyes, rubbing your hands together until they are warm, placing them over your eyes, and holding them there.
- See if you can feel the warmth in your eyes.
- Take a few breaths in this position.

YOGA FOR BED BOUND ELDERS

Deep Breathing (3-Part, Diaphragmatic)

This yogic breathing practice serves many purposes and may be practiced by almost anyone who can follow simple instructions. For those with physical limitations, it may be modified.

- Lying on your back in a comfortable position, place both hands on your belly. You may want to close your eyes. Let your belly be soft and begin to take some nice deep breaths in through your nose, if possible. Feel the breath expand your belly on the inhalation, and as you exhale, feel your belly deflate. Let the breaths be deep and slow.
- Place the hands on your ribs and fill them as you inhale. Feel your ribs expand and contract with the in and out breaths. Breathe in and out as slowly and deeply as possible.
- Put your fingers just below your collarbone and feel the inhale and exhale in this area.

Now, put all three breaths together for three-part breathing—breathing into the belly, then the ribs, and then the upper chest, exhaling in the opposite order. Count slowly as you breathe in and out, extending the length of the breath as long as possible. See if you can make your exhalation at least as long as your inhalation.

Bed Stretches

For each of the following, the person is guided to move gently and slowly and to pay attention to the process of moving as well as to holding a position. Paying attention to breathing, during and between the movements, is integral to movement meditation.

- Turn the head from side to side, looking over the shoulder.
- Look up and look down.
- Roll shoulders forward and backward.
- Extend arms to sides, shoulder height, and stretch hands out.
- Reach up as high as possible and stretch you entire body from fingers to toes. Become aware of all your joints and stretch through the joints.
- Lift knees, one at a time.
- Extend calves and feet, one at a time, rolling feet in and then out.

APPENDIX B

Guided Meditations

Below are meditations you may wish to practice. They are presented as if I were guiding you. Practice them yourself. It will be simpler to practice these meditations listening rather than reading, so you may record yourself reading this or purchase CDs. There are many versions of these practices available on CD or in yoga and meditation classes. (See suggested resources below under Spirituality and Healing Resources, Web Sites.) Experience a variety of teachers and find what suits you best. When offering guidance to others, adapt to the population. Make them your own.

BREATH AWARENESS

Paying attention to our breath is the most basic, simple, and yet challenging practice. We always can come back to our breath, using it as an anchor in the sea of life.

- Focus your attention on your breath, let the breath be, without directing it in any way. Note how it feels in your body to sit here and breathe.
- It may be helpful to find one area of your body to focus on. You may, for example, focus your attention on the area around the nostrils where the breath enters and exits. You might notice the sensation of breath on your upper lip or nostrils. Or you may want to focus your attention on the belly or chest, noticing the gentle rise and fall with the in and out breath.
- Not changing or manipulating your breath, simply letting it be. Notice and observe. What is your breath like right now? Is it short or long, deep or shallow, fast or slow, even or ragged? More than thinking about your breath, be *with* your breath.

- Sometimes, you may notice that it is difficult to stay focused on the breath. You may find that your mind has wandered into thoughts. This is very normal. When you notice that your attention has wandered, bring it back, without self-judgment or criticism.
- Sit quietly for a while, simply observing your breath. If you need to move or adjust your posture, do so mindfully, with awareness. Notice all the sensations connected with moving your body.

BODY SCAN

The body scan is a slow, detailed awareness of body sensations, often starting from the toes and gradually working one's way up to the top of the head. This practice may be done sitting or lying down or lying down on your back. During the body scan, you may notice that your mind has wandered. When you notice it, return your awareness to wherever we are in the exercise at that moment. You may also notice areas that are painful, and other areas in which you do not experience any sensations. Observe them all.

- Begin by turning your attention to your feet resting flat on the ground. Without moving them, notice any physical sensations in your feet as they rest here. Perhaps you have removed your shoes and can feel the floor cool on your soles, or perhaps you have your shoes on and can feel them wrapping your feet. If you are lying down, you may feel the pressure of your heels on the floor. Notice the toes, arch, top and bottom, and sides of the feet. If it feels right to you, direct your breath all the way down into the feet as you breathe in, and as you breathe out, breathe all the way out from the feet.
- Expand your awareness to include your ankles, left and right. You may want to imagine you are breathing in and out from your ankles.
- Next, spread the focus of your attention to your lower legs or calves. Notice your skin, your bones, your muscles. Notice any physical sensation, perhaps tingling, throbbing, warmth, or coolness. Or a lack of sensations.
- Move your awareness up to include your knees. The knee is a complicated joint that serves us well as we walk, sit, and stand throughout the day. Breathe into your knees and breathe out of your knees.
- When you are ready, expand your focus to include your thighs. Perhaps feeling the pressure of the thighs on the chair or your hands on the lap. Note the top, sides, and bottom of the thighs and any physical sensations or lack of sensation. What does it feel like to have no sensation,

if this is the case? Inhale into your thighs and exhale out from your thighs.

- Take your attention to your buttocks as they rest in the chair or on the floor. Include the pelvis. Notice any sensations in this area or lack of sensation. Breathe into the pelvis and buttocks and breathe out from the pelvis and buttocks.
- Bring your awareness to include your back, the lower back, middle, and upper. You may notice areas of tension, pain, or stress in your back. Note them as you breathe in and out of your entire back area. If there is tension or pain, what does it feel like? Can you observe the sensations as they rise and fall, come and go? Can you feel the expansion and contraction of the back ribs with your inhalation and exhalation? Breathe into the back and out from your entire back.
- Turn your attention to the front of your torso, including your belly, your front ribs, and your chest. Note, if you can, where you feel your breath. See if you can become aware of your internal organs, your lungs, heart, intestines, all the organs that support you every day. We often do not think of our wonderful body until we have illness or pain. Can you just observe your body as you sit or lie here, breathing?
- Now, focus your attention on your arms. Bring your awareness all the way down to the fingers. Direct your breath all the way down with an inhalation and all the way up with an exhalation. Notice any sensations: tingling, throbbing, itching, moisture. Notice your palms, the top of your hands, and your wrists. Notice your hands at rest.
- Move your awareness to your shoulders and neck, areas where many experience tension as they "carry the world." Let your neck and shoulders be as they are for now, noticing any sensations.
- As you bring attention to your throat, can you feel your breath as it travels from your mouth or nose to your lungs?
- Bring your attention up to your head. At the back of your head, the scalp area, notice any and all sensations or lack of sensations. Maybe you notice tingling, itching, warmth or coolness. Or not, simply notice.
- Move your attention to your face. Start with your jaw, the bone and the joint attaching your jaw to your skull. Are your teeth clenched? Notice your teeth, your tongue, and your lips. Now focus on your cheeks, your nose, your nostrils, and the area below your nostrils. You may notice your breath, entering cool, exiting warm. Turn your attention to your eyes and the area around your eyes: your eyeballs resting in the sockets, your eyebrows. And finally, your forehead. Breathe into your entire face and breathe out from your entire face.

- Now, imagine that there is a hole at the very top of your skull, at the place where you had a soft spot as an infant. And imagine your breath could enter through this spot. As you breathe in, imagine your breath can travel all the way through your head, neck, torso, arms, and legs, all the way down to your feet. On the out breath, imagine the breath travels up from your feet through your entire body and out through the spot at the top of your head.
- After a few of these directed breaths, let your breath to return to normal, without controlling it in any way. Take a few more moments to note sensations you are feeling right here and now, and where you are feeling them. You may also want to observe feelings and thoughts that arise. Rather than attending your body, part by part, take a few moments to observe your body as a whole. You may feel different even after a short exercise such as this. If it is the case, know that you can always use your breath as tool to bring you back to the present moment.
- As the meditation draws to an end, allow your breath to deepen slightly. Slowly awaken the body to movement, moving your fingers or toes in any way you like. As you resume activity, remember that we all have the capacity to enter a space of healing and growth within us, at any moment, simply by paying attention to our breath and our body.

A more in-depth discussion of the body scan can be found in the following source: J. Kabat-Zinn, *Full Catastrophe Living: Using the Wisdom of Your Body and Mind to Face Stress, Pain and Illness* (New York: Dell, 1990), pp. 75–93.

FORGIVENESS MEDITATION

Introducing the meditation:

Forgiveness does not justify or condone hurtful behavior.

Forgiving others and ourselves is something that we do for ourselves so that we do not have to carry the pain any longer.

It is a process that can take some time.

It is something we do for its own sake; we do not have to share it with others.

If you are not sure, try it and see if you feel better!

Throughout the meditation, do only what feels right to you; listen to your inner voice.

Begin by sitting or lying in a comfortable position.

Initially, focus on your breath.

When you feel ready, think of someone you have hurt, betrayed, abandoned, or caused suffering to, knowingly or unknowingly, in word, deed, or thought, out of your own pain, fear, and suffering. And ask forgiveness of him or her [it could be yourself!].

Now, think of ways you have betrayed, hurt, or abandoned your beautiful self in words, deeds, actions, or thoughts, out of fear, pain, and suffering. Extend a full and heartfelt forgiveness.

Finally, if you feel comfortable with it, think of someone who has wounded, betrayed, or abandoned you, knowingly or unknowingly, out of his or her own pain, fear, and suffering. If you can, bring that person to your mind's eye. To the extent that you are ready to, send forgiveness to that person, releasing your anger and pain.

(Excerpted from a longer forgiveness meditation by Beth Roth. A CD of the full Forgiveness Meditation is available at http://www.newhavenweb.com/bethroth.)

APPENDIX C

Aromatherapy

Aromatherapy is the use of essential oils that are extracted from plants and distilled for their therapeutic properties. Chapter 3 discusses aromatherapy, safety precautions, and five essential oils. This appendix offers a few more ideas and some specific directions for using essential oils in the nursing home.

SAFETY REMINDERS

Essential oils tend to be mild and rarely cause a reaction. Caution and common sense is still advised, especially in working with elders. For this reason, I will repeat some of the precautions. Aromatherapy is best used in conjunction with medical treatment; it is not a replacement for qualified medical care. A doctor or nurse should always be consulted. Talk with an aromatherapist when possible. Make sure all staff who will be using the essential oils are trained in safety measures. Discontinue use of the essential oil if the elder, or anyone, starts coughing or complaining. If the elder's skin is broken, do not use the oils on the skin. A skin patch test is always a good idea.

Skin Patch Test

Dilute the essential oil you want to test in a carrier oil, such as almond oil, and place a drop on the elder's forearm. Loosely cover the area and wait 24 hours. Check the patch for any redness.

Material Safety Data Sheet (MSDS)

The Material Safety Data Sheet is available for essential oils and can help you further determine safety and emergency treatment. MSDS information is available on the Internet. The following site is one of many that have basic safety information and links for MSDSs on essential oils: http://www.mountainroseherbs.com/newsletter/essential_oils_handle_with_care.php

SUGGESTED USES IN THE NURSING HOME

Bath

Put 10–13 drops of an essential oil (lavender is good for elders) in a full tub of water. If you put the essential oil in while the bath is running, the aroma will fill the room.

Sleeping Environment

Put one drop on the bed pillow, in an area that will not come into contact with the elder's face. Lavender is good for relaxation and sleep. Alternately, a diffuser can be placed in the elder's room. The diffuser must not be accessible to the elder, however, since the resident may not be supervised at all times.

Hallways

Diffusers can be used in hallways to cover a large area. A combination of essential oils using lemongrass, lavender, and geranium is a balancing blend.

Dining Areas

Elders may benefit from the use of cinnamon oil in the dining area as an appetite stimulant. A diffuser can be used or a plain spray water bottle. Use 5 drops per 1 ounce of water, and spritz the room.

Individual Applications

There are a number of ways that aromatherapy can be individually utilized. One drop on a cotton ball can be waved under the nose of the elder, or 2 to 3 drops can be put on clothing, again in an area that would not be in contact with the skin. For massages, use 5 drops of an essential oil in a carrier oil such as almond, grapeseed, or jojoba. *Never apply any essential oil directly onto an elder's skin.* Remember to check the MSDS, and do not use peppermint or cinnamon, even diluted, on an elder's skin.

HOW TO USE ESSENTIAL OILS

Using moderation is always a good idea for essential oils. The effects are subtle and individual. Proceed slowly when considering the amounts to use and the length of time. You may want to start using one essential oil. Lavender is the best researched and utilized. Become familiar with the recommended applications and safety measures. Essential oils may be purchased at your health food store or via the Internet at the Web sites suggested in Appendix F. Make sure you are using a pure essential oil from a reputable company. It will cost a little more, but it will be worth it. One great way to start using essential oils is to try them yourself at home or in your office.

MASSAGE

Aromatherapy Massage Oil

Essential oils are applied topically mixed with a carrier oil. The carrier oil can be 100% pure jojoba oil or almond oil, which can be purchased at most health food stores. A 1% dilution is desirable for elders. Measure 1 ounce of almond oil or jojoba oil (approximately 300 ccs), and place 5 drops of an essential oil into the mixture. Shake the bottle well before using. Remember, certain oils, like cinnamon, are not to be used on skin even when they are diluted because they are skin irritants. Read labels carefully.

Hand Massage

Hand massages offer many benefits for the giver and the receiver. A hand massage often naturally flows from the hand holding that many elders enjoy. It is important to start slowly and to ask the elders if they would like a hand massage. If they cannot verbally respond, it is especially important to watch for nonverbal cues. With clean hands, pour a small amount of the oil (if you are using oil), about the size of a quarter, into the palm of your hand. Rub your hands together to warm them and the oil. Both you and the elder should be seated, and it is most comfortable if the elder's arm is supported so that he or she can relax. Hold one of the elder's hands in both of yours. Begin massaging the back of the hand in light, slow circular movements. The pressure should be about 3 on a scale of 1–10. Massage each of the fingers and the joints, again in slow circular movements. Turn the elder's hand over and massage the palm and wrist. Again turning the hand over, gently stroke the lower arm if it is available. The whole hand should take 4–7 minutes. When you have finished one hand, pat it with a towel to remove excess oil and start on the other hand. You may find yourself relaxed also by the essential oils and the rhythmic touch.

I have found most elders to be very receptive to hand massages. For some, it is the last available form of communication. Others are not so receptive or prefer a hand rub without oil. I have also noticed how tense many elders hands are and how they often relax noticeably following a hand massage. As always, when working with confused elders, exercise caution in case the elder becomes very upset and physically agitated.

Shoulder Massage

Most elders really enjoy shoulder rubs. They are a great way to end a group. As elders are sitting, I go around behind the circle. Before touching the elder, I ask permission. Then I place my hands gently on their shoulders. The massage should be very gentle, and elders should always be asked along the way if the pressure is good. Sometimes, I am massaging gently, I think, and the elder will say it is too strong. Sometimes, I will just lay my hands on the elder's shoulder, neck, or head and send warmth. If it seems OK, I end with a hug.

Brief Stress Reduction Session Ideas

As described in Chapter 12, using shorter sessions on the nursing units maximizes staff participation. A monthly theme can be helpful in focusing ideas and resources for brief stress reduction programs. Themes can be based on the needs of your population as ascertained by an initial survey. The most helpful brief classes are experiential and include handouts and referrals. Some of the programs we offered were:

- Mindfulness-based stress reduction
- Chair yoga and breathing exercises
- Self-massage
- Coping with chronic pain
- Healthy eating
- Mood management
- Aromatherapy (A. Lombardo, personal communication, August 30, 2007)

The Web can be an excellent resource for information on all of these topics. In brief sessions, the instructor's presence is essential, as these sessions tend to be full of challenges such as interruptions, noise, and other distractions.

Handouts for Staff Stress Reduction

HANDOUT #1: 21 WAYS TO REDUCE STRESS DURING THE WORKDAY

1. Take a few minutes in the morning to be quiet and meditate. Sit or lie down and be with yourself . . . gaze out the window, listen to the sounds of nature, or take a slow, quiet walk.

2. While waiting for the elevator or your train or bus, take a minute to quietly pay attention to your breathing.

3. While riding the bus, subway, or taxi to work, become aware of body tension, for example, shoulders raised, stomach tight, hands clenched. Consciously work at releasing, dissolving that tension.

4. Decide whether to listen to music or the news, read, or just be by yourself, paying attention.

5. While walking, notice the physical sensations.

6. Notice your breath or the sky while waiting for a light to change.

7. Before arriving at your workplace, take a moment to orient yourself to your workday.

8. While sitting at your desk, keyboard, etc., monitor your bodily sensations and tension levels and consciously attempt to let go of excess tension.

9. Use your breaks to truly relax rather than simply to "pause." For example, instead of having a cigarette or coffee, take a 2- or 5-minute walk, or sit at your desk and stretch or meditate.

10. At lunch, changing your environment can be helpful.

11. Close your door (if you have one), and take some time to consciously relax.

---

12. Decide to "stop" for 1 to 3 minutes every hour during the workday. Become aware of your breathing and bodily sensations. Use it as a time to regroup and recoup.

13. Use everyday clues in your environment as reminders to "center" yourself, for example, the telephone ringing, turning on the computer, etc.

14. Take some time at lunch or break to share with close associates. Choose topics not necessarily work-related.

15. Choose to eat one or two lunches per week in silence. Use it as time to eat slowly and to be with yourself.

16. At the end of a workday, retrace your activities of the day, acknowledging and congratulating yourself for what you've accomplished and make a list for tomorrow.

17. As you leave work, pay attention to your walking: the feeling of cold or warmth on your body. Try to accept it rather than resist it. Listen to the sounds outside the office. Can you walk without feeling rushed?

18. Walk home once or twice a week, or if it is too far, walk an extra stop or two before you get on the subway or bus.

19. While walking, notice if you are rushing. What does it feel like? What can you do about it? Remember, you have more control than you imagine.

20. Before you enter your building, take a moment to come back to the present. Orient yourself to being home and with your household members.

21. Change out of your work clothes when you get home; it helps you to make a smoother transition into your "role." You can spare the 5 minutes to do this. Center yourself, and, if possible, take 5 or 10 minutes to be quiet and still.

Adapted for city dwellers from the following source: Santorelli, S. F. (1996). Mindfulness and mastery in the workplace: 21 ways to reduce stress during the workday. In A. Kotler (Ed.), Engaged Buddhist reader *(pp. 39–46). Fitchburg, MA: Parallax.*

HANDOUT #2: BASIC PRINCIPLES FOR SETTING UP DAILY HATHA YOGA/MINDFULNESS STRESS MANAGEMENT PRACTICE

- Build with simplicity; keep it simple and direct. Make one or two small changes in your daily routine, practice them until they become habits.

- Don't try to change the world or yourself in a day. Make a reasonable time commitment. You earn depending on what you invest. Find a commitment you can keep.
- Consistency is important. A 5-minute commitment done consistently will provide real benefits, whereas an hour done haphazardly will lead to little skill development (e.g., learning to play an instrument).
- Persist until the habit of skill is established. If the small tasks are finished, the will is strengthened. On the other hand, if self-assigned tasks are left unfinished, the will is subtly weakened.
- Build a strong foundation and continue. Build skills at relaxation, one part at a time.
- Be playful, experiment with the practices. Don't be afraid to try new ways of gaining insight, developing interests, and solving problems.

Courtesy of Luis F. Sierra, ADK Yoga, www.adkyoga.com

Daily Stress Management Routines

If You Have 6 to 12 Minutes Daily

- A.M.: When you wake up in the morning, while still lying in bed, do a few rounds of diaphragmatic breathing (2–4 minutes).
- Midday: During lunch break, take a few minutes (2–4 minutes) to do some deep breathing or observe the body, breath, and mind.
- P.M.: At the end of the day, at home do some gentle stretching (2–4 minutes) before doing other tasks, having dinner, or going out.

If You Have 15 to 20 Minutes Daily

- A.M.: When you wake up, sit up in bed supported by a pillow or bed covers, breathe deeply, leading into diaphragmatic breathing or the three-part breath as described in class (2–4 minutes).
- Midday: Stretch the body while breathing comfortably; do a forward bend, a standing stretch (3–4 minutes). Then, close your eyes and observe the breath (2–3 minutes).
- P.M.: Before having dinner, stretch the body for a few minutes, followed by a breath awareness exercise (4 minutes). Instead of watching TV or reading, do a brief meditation before going to sleep (4–5 minutes).

If You Have 30 to 45 Minutes Daily

- A.M.: Before eating breakfast, stretch the body for a few minutes, and then observe the breath, gradually deepening it, eventually doing a few rounds of three-part, yoga breath and/or any other breathing exercise you are comfortable with (5–10 minutes).
- Midday: Before eating lunch, close the eyes and observe the breath, followed by a period of meditation (5–10 minutes).
- P.M.: Before having dinner (it can be done in a gym if there is a quiet room or a place where there aren't too many distractions), do deep breathing and stretches (8–10 minutes), a deep relaxation (5–8 minutes), and a breathing practice and meditation (5 minutes). Before going to sleep, do a brief meditation (2–4 minutes).

Be creative, develop your own routine, and find what works best for you, given your schedule and interests.

Courtesy of Luis F. Sierra, ADK Yoga, www.adkyoga.com

HANDOUT #3: MINI RELAXATION EXERCISES

- Mini relaxation exercises are focused breathing techniques that help reduce anxiety and tension immediately.
- You can do them with your eyes open or closed (but make sure that your eyes are open while you are driving!).
- You can do them any place, at any time; no one will know that you are doing them.

Ways to Do a Mini

Try to make the breath a belly breath or a diaphragmatic breath. If that isn't comfortable, then breathe in through the nose and exhale through the mouth, or just breathe deeply in whatever way is comfortable. A good way to practice the belly breathing is to lie on your back and place a hand on the abdomen or belly, feeling that as you inhale the hand moves up as the belly expands and then the hand goes down as you exhale. Keep the stomach muscles relaxed. If you feel lightheaded or dizzy, return to a regular comfortable breath.

Mini Version One

Count very slowly silently to yourself from 10 down to 1, one number for each full breath (an inhalation and an exhalation). For example, with the first deep breath count "ten," the next breath count "nine," . . . etc. When you get to "one," go back to "ten." Do this for a few rounds and then notice how you feel. If it feels comfortable, do it for as long as you like.

Mini Version Two

As you inhale, count very slowly up to four; as you exhale, count slowly back down to one. Thus, as you inhale, you say to yourself, "one, two, three, four"; as you exhale, you say to yourself, "four, three, two, one." Do this several times.

Mini Version Three

After each inhalation, pause a few seconds, saying silently to yourself "in." And then as you exhale, pause for a few seconds, saying silently to yourself "out." Do this for several breaths.

Good Times to Do a Mini

- While stuck in traffic
- When put on hold during an important phone call
- While waiting in your doctor's waiting room
- When someone says something that bothers you
- At all red lights
- When waiting for a phone call
- In the dentist's chair
- When you feel overwhelmed by what you need to accomplish in the near future
- While standing in line
- When in pain

THE ONLY TIME THAT MINIS DO NOT WORK IS WHEN YOU FORGET TO DO THEM!!!

So, go do a mini!

Courtesy of Luis F. Sierra, ADK Yoga, www.adkyoga.com

Midway Review

How am I finding the course so far?

Any problems/difficulties with

Body scan

Yoga

Meditation

Am I solving the problems?

Things I am learning about myself?

Am I making time to practice?

Any comments, suggestions, requests?

Name (optional)

Beth Roth, personal communication, October 10, 2000.

For staff classes we also provided information on chair/office yoga with photos and included a brief resource list of books on stress reduction, sources for stress reduction tapes, and local stores that sold stress reduction tapes and books as well as aromatherapy shops.

APPENDIX F

Selected Bibliography
and Web Sites

MINDFULNESS AND MEDITATION RESOURCES

Books

Baer, R. A. (Ed.). (2006). *Mindfulness based treatment approaches: Clinician's guide to evidence base and applications.* Amsterdam: Academic.

Begley, S. (2007). *Train your mind, change your brain: How a new science reveals our extraordinary potential to transform ourselves.* New York: Ballantine.

Hayes, S. C. (2005). *Get out of your mind and into your life: The new acceptance and commitment therapy.* Oakland, CA: New Harbinger.

Hayes, S. C., Strosahl, K. D., & Wilson, K. G. (2003). *Acceptance and commitment therapy: An experiential approach to behavior change.* New York: Guilford.

Kabat-Zinn, J. (1990). *Full catastrophe living: Using the wisdom of your body and mind to face stress, pain and illness.* New York: Dell.

Kabat-Zinn, J. (1994). *Wherever you go, there you are: Mindfulness meditation in everyday life.* New York: Hyperion.

Kabat-Zinn, J. (2005). *Coming to our senses: Healing ourselves and the world through mindfulness.* New York: Hyperion.

Kornfield, J. (1993). *A path with heart: A guide through the perils and promises of spiritual life.* New York: Bantam.

Kramer, G. (2007). *Insight dialogue: The interpersonal path to freedom.* Boston: Shambhala.

Linehan, M. (1993). *Skills training manual for treating borderline personality disorder.* New York: Guilford.

Nhat Hanh, T. (1987). *The miracle of mindfulness.* Boston: Beacon.

Nhat Hanh, T. (1991). *Peace is every step.* New York: Bantam.

Nhat Hanh, T. (2002). *No death, no fear.* New York: Riverhead.

Rosenbaum, E. (2005). *Here for now: Living well with cancer through mindfulness.* Hardwick, MA: Satya House.

Santorelli, S. (1999). *Heal thy self.* New York: Bell Tower.

Segal, Z. V., Willams, J. M. G., & Teasdale, J. D. (2002). *Mindfulness-based cognitive therapy for depression: A new approach to preventing relapse.* New York: Guilford.

Siegel, D. J. (2007). *The mindful brain.* New York: W. W. Norton.

Articles

Astin, J. A. (1997). Stress reduction through mindfulness meditation. *Psychotherapy Psychosometric, 66,* 97–106.

Davidson, R. J., Kabat-Zinn, J., Schumacher, J., Rosenkranz, M., Muller, D., Santorelli, S. F., et al. (2003). Alterations in brain and immune function produced by mindfulness meditation. *Psychosomatic Medicine, 65,* 564–570.

Epstein, R. M. (1999). Mindful practice. *Journal of the American Medical Association, 282*(9), 833–839.

Kabat-Zinn, J. (1982). An outpatient program in behavioral medicine for chronic pain patients based on the practice of mindfulness meditation. *General Hospital Psychiatry, 4,* 33–47.

Kabat-Zinn, J., Lipworth, L., Burney, R., & Sellers, W. (1986). Four-year follow-up of a meditation-based program for the self-regulation of chronic pain: treatment outcomes and compliance. *Clinical Journal of Pain, 2*(3), 159–174.

Kabat-Zinn, J., Massion, A. O., Kristeller, J., Peterson, L. G., Fletcher, K. E., Pbert, L., Lenderking, W. R., & Santorelli, S. F. et al. (1992). Effectiveness of a meditation-based program in the treatment of anxiety disorders. *American Journal of Psychiatry, 149*(7), 936–943.

Lantz, M. S., Buchalter, E. N., & McBee, L. (1997). The Wellness Group: A novel intervention for coping with disruptive behavior in elderly nursing home residents. *The Gerontologist, 37*(4), 551–556.

McBee, L. (2004). Mindfulness practice with the frail elderly and their caregivers: Changing the practitioner-patient relationship. *Topics in Geriatric Rehabilitation, 19*(4), 257–264.

McBee, L., Westreich, L., & Likourezos, A. (2004). A psychoeducational relaxation group for pain and stress management in the nursing home. *Journal of Social Work in Long-Term Care, 3*(1), 15–28.

Roth, B., & Stanley, T.-W. (2002a). Mindfulness-based stress reduction and healthcare in the inner city: Preliminary findings. *Alternative Therapies, 8*(1), 60–67.

Roth, B., & Stanley, T.-W. (2002b). Mindfulness-based stress reduction and healthcare utilization in the inner city: preliminary findings. *Alternative Therapies in Health Medicine, 8*(1), 60–62, 64–66.

Schmidt, S. (2004). Mindfulness and healing intention: Concepts, practice, and research evaluation. *The Journal of Alternative and Complementary Medicine, 10*(Supplement 1), S-7–S-14.

Shalek, M., & Doyle, S. (1998). Relaxation revisited: An adaptation of a relaxation group geared toward geriatrics with behavior problems. *American Journal of Alzheimer's Disease and Other Dementias, 13*(3), 160–162.

Smith, A. (2004). Clinical uses of mindfulness training for older people. *Behavioral and Cognitive Psychotherapy, 32,* 423–430.

Speca, M., Carlson, L. E., Goodey, E., & Angen, M. (2000). A randomized, wait-list controlled clinical trial: The effect of a mindfulness meditation-based stress reduction program on mood and symptoms of stress in cancer programs. *Psychosometric Medicine, 62*(5), 613–622.

Web Sites

Interpersonal meditation practice: Insight Dialogue—mindfulness in relationship information and training. http://www.metta.org/
Mindfulness-based CDs in English and Spanish: Forgiveness meditation. http://www.newhavenweb.com/bethroth
Mindfulness-Based Stress Reduction: The Center for Mindfulness in Medicine, Health Care and Society—information and training resources. http://www.umassmed.edu/cfm/

YOGA RESOURCES

Books

Bell, L., & Seyfer, E. (2000). *Gentle yoga: A guide to low-impact exercise.* Berkeley, CA: Celestial Arts.
Boccio, F. J. (2004). *Mindfulness yoga: The awakened union of breath, body, and mind,* Somerville, MA: Wisdom.
Cappy, P. (2006). *Yoga for all of us: A modified series of traditional poses for any age and ability.* New York: St. Martin's.
Christensen, A. (1999). *American Yoga Association's easy does it yoga: The safe and gentle way to health and well-being.* New York: Fireside.
Paul, R. (2004). *The yoga of sound.* Novato, CA: New World Library.

Web Sites

Silver Age Yoga: Offers online and in-person training in yoga for elders for certified yoga teachers. http://www.silverageyoga.org/

COMPLEMENTARY AND ALTERNATIVE RESOURCES

Books

Cousins, N. (2005). *Anatomy of an illness.* New York: W. W. Norton.
Farhi, D. (1996). *The breathing book: Good health and vitality through essential breath work.* New York: Henry Holt.
Fisher, P. P. (1995). *More than movement for fit to frail older adults: Creative activities for the body, mind, and spirit.* Baltimore: Health Professionals.
Institute of Medicine of the National Academies. (2005). *Complementary and alternative medicine in the United States.* Washington, DC: National Academies Press.

Mackenzie, E. R., & Rakel, B. (Eds.). (2006). *Complementary and alternative medicine for older adults.* New York: Springer.

Oz, M., with Arias, R., & Oz, L. (1999). *Healing from the heart.* New York: Plume.

Reynolds, R. A. (1995). *Bring me the ocean: Nature as teacher, messenger, and intermediary.* Acton, MA: VanderWyk & Burnham.

Sapolsky, R. (2004). *Why zebras don't get ulcers.* New York: Owl.

Articles

Grzywacz, J. G., Suerken, C. K., Quandt, S. A., Bell, R. A., Lang, W., & Arcury, T. A. (2006). Older adults' use of complementary and alternative medicine for mental health: Findings from the 2002 National Health Interview Study. *The Journal of Alternative and Complementary Medicine, 12*(5), 467–473.

HPNA Board of Directors. (2003). HPNA Position Paper: Complementary therapies. *Journal of Hospice and Palliative Nursing, 5*(2), 113–117.

Kolcaba, K., Dowd, T., Steiner, R., & Mitzel, A. (2004). Efficacy of hand massage for enhancing the comfort of hospice patients. *Journal of Hospice and Palliative Nursing, 6*(2), 91–101.

Lindberg, D. A. (2005). Integrative review of research related to meditation, spirituality, and the elderly. *Geriatric Nursing. 26*(6), 372–377.

Ness, J., Cirillo, D. J., Weir, D. R., Nisly, N. L., & Wallace, R. B. (2005). Use of complementary medicine in older Americans: Results from the retirement study. *The Gerontologist, 45*(4), 516–524.

Tilden, V. P., Drach, L. L., & Tolle, S. W. (2004) Complementary and alternative therapy use at end-of-life in community settings. *The Journal of Alternative and Complementary Medicine, 10*(5), 811–817.

Wolsko, P. M., Eisenberg, D. M., Davis, R. B., & Phillips, R. S. (2004). Use of mind-body therapies: Results of a national survey. *Journal of General Internal Medicine, 19,* 43–50.

Web Sites

Laughter Yoga Clubs: Dr. Madan Kataria initiated these 11 years ago, now practiced worldwide. http://www.laughteryoga.org/

"M" massage technique and aromatherapy. www.rjbuckle.com

National Institute of Health: Complementary and Alternative Medicine. http://nccam.nih.gov/news/camsurvey_fs1.htm#use

The Touch Research Institute: Studies the effects of touch therapy. http://www6.miami.edu/touch-research/

SPIRITUALITY AND HEALING RESOURCES

Books

Chodron, P. (1997). *When things fall apart.* Boston: Shambhala.

Dass, R. (2000). *Still here.* New York: Riverhead.

Gawain, S. (1991). *Meditations: Creative visualization and meditation exercises to enrich your life.* Novato, CA: Nataraj.

Goldstein, J. (1993). *Insight meditation: The practice of freedom.* Boston: Shambhala.

Kearney, M. (2000). *A place of healing: Working with suffering in living and dying.* Oxford, UK: Oxford University.

Levine, S. (1987). *Healing into life and death.* New York: Anchor.

Levine, S. (1991). *Guided meditations, explorations and healings.* New York: Anchor.

Lozoff, B. (1985). *We're all doing time: A guide for getting free.* Durham, NC: Hanuman Foundation.

Luskin, F. (2003). *Forgive for good: Proven prescription for health and happiness.* San Francisco: Harper.

Mindell, A. (1989). *Coma: The dreambody near death.* London: Penguin.

Naperstek, B. (1994). *Staying well with guided imagery.* New York: Warner.

Remen, R. N. (1996). *Kitchen table wisdom.* New York: Riverhead.

Rinpoche, S. (1992). *The Tibetan book of living and dying.* (P. Gaffney & A. Harvey, Eds.). San Francisco: HarperSanFrancisco.

Rosenberg, L. (1998). *Breath by breath.* Boston: Shambhala.

Salzberg, S. (1995). *Loving-kindness.* Boston: Shambhala.

Thera, N., & Bodhi, B. (Trans. & Eds.). (1999). *Numerical discourses of the Buddha: An anthology of Suttas from the Anguttara Nikaya.* Walnut Creek, CA: AltaMira.

Web Sites

Belleruth Naparstek: Guided imagery CDs. http://www.healthjourneys.com/

Shambhala Press: Books and CDs with an emphasis on spiritual practices and traditions. http://www.shambhala.com/

Sounds True: CDs and tapes from a variety of spiritual and healing traditions. www.soundstrue.com

AROMATHERAPY RESOURCES

Books

Lawless, J. (1995). *The illustrated encyclopedia of essential oils.* Rockport, MD: Element.

Price, S., & Price, L. (1999). *Aromatherapy for health professionals.* London: Churchill and Livingstone.

Tisserand, R., & Balacs, T. (1995). *Essential oil safety: A guide for health care professionals.* London: Churchill and Livingstone.

Worwood, V. A. (1991). *The complete book of essential oils and aromatherapy.* Novato, CA: New World Library.

Web Sites

For essential oils, look in health food stores for those in *dark bottles* with the *Latin name* on the bottle. There are no regulations on these products, and much of what is called aromatherapy is not a pure essential oil.

Aroma Therapeutix: Supplies: essential oils, diffusers, perfume sticks, paper pyramids, and other related items. http://www.aromatherapeutix.com/1-800-308-6284.

Aromaweb: Online information on aromatherapy. www.aromaweb.com

Mountain Rose Herbs: Basic safety information and links for MSDS sheets on essential oils. http://www.mountainroseherbs.com/newsletter/essential_oils_handle_with_care.php

The National Association for Holistic Aromatherapy: http://www.naha.org/888-ASK-NAHA or (206) 547-2164.

Young Living Essential Oils: Supplies essential oils, diffusers, and other related items. http://www.youngliving.us

ELDERS, CAREGIVERS, AND MODELS OF CARE RESOURCES

Books

Bell, V., & Troxel, D. (2003). *The best friend's approach to Alzheimer's care.* Baltimore: Health Professionals.

Feil, N. (2002). *The validation breakthrough* (2nd ed.). Baltimore: Health Professionals.

Fisher, P. P. (1995). *More than movement for fit to frail older adults: Creative activities for the body, mind, and spirit.* Baltimore: Health Professionals.

Ronch, J., & Goldfield, J. (Eds.). (2002). *Mental wellness in aging: Strength-based approaches.* Baltimore: Health Professionals.

Schachter-Shalomi, Z., & Miller, R. (1995). *From age-ing to sage-ing: A profound new vision of growing older.* New York: Warner.

Spink, K. (2006). *The miracle, the message, the story: Jean Vanier and l'Arche.* London: Hidden Spring.

Thomas, W. H. (2004). *What are old people for? How elders will save the world.* Acton, MA: VanderWyk & Burnham.

Toseland, R. W. (1995). *Group work with the elderly and family caregivers.* New York: Springer.

Weiner, A. S., & Ronch, J. L. (2003). *Culture change in long term care.* Binghamton, NY: Haworth.

Web Sites

The Eden Alternative: Seeking to remake the experience of aging around the world, including deinstitutionalizing the culture and environment of today's nursing homes and other long-term care institutions. http://www.edenalt.org/

Family Caregiver Alliance: Offers information, services, and publications based on caregiver needs at local, state, and national levels. www.caregiver.org

L'Arche Communities: Founded by Jean Vanier in France in 1964, they bring together people, some with developmental disabilities and some without, who choose to share their lives by living together in faith-based communities. http://www.larcheusa.org/.

Live Oak: Dedicated to transforming the places where elders live, the services they receive and provide. http://liveoakinstitute.org/home.html

Paraprofessional Healthcare Institute: Works to improve the lives of people who need home and residential care—and the lives of the workers who provide that care. http://www.paraprofessional.org/

The Pioneer Network: A connecting organization that promotes grassroots activities and new ways of deinstitutionalizing services and individualizing care across the aging services spectrum. http://www.pioneernetwork.net/

POETRY RESOURCES

Poetry can provide another voice for mindfulness. Poems are about paying attention and seeing things in new ways. Below are listed a few poetry books. One easy way to discover and enjoy new poems is to listen to the Writer's Almanac on National Public Radio. If you sign up to receive it on your e-mail at http://writers almanac.publicradio.org/, you will receive a poem each day!

Berry, W. (1998). *The selected poems of Wendell Berry.* Washington, DC: Counterpoint.

Oliver, M. (2005). *New and selected poems: Volume Two.* Boston: Beacon.

Oliver, M. (2006). *Thirst: Poems.* Boston: Beacon.

Rumi. (Barks, C., with Moyne, J., Trans.). (1995). *The essential Rumi.* San Francisco: HarperSanFrancisco.

Walcott, D. (1986). *Collected poems 1948–1984.* New York: Farrar, Straus & Giroux.

For Guided Meditation CDs, further publication listings and other information contact Lucia McBee, www.luciamcbee.com

Index

Acute care, 5, 11
Aging, 163
  conscious, 164, 165
  meditation on, 86
  models of, 164–165
  of population, 5, 109
Alms-houses, 6
Alternative medical systems, 7
Alzheimer's Association, 73
Alzheimer's disease, 72. *See also*
  Dementia
Anger
  in MBEC informal caregiver
  groups, 132
  in MBEC professional caregivers
  course, 141–142
L'Arche, 166, 167, 168
Aromatherapy, 7, 33–34, 38. *See also*
  Essential oils
  applications of, 35–36, 188–190
  as CAM dementia intervention, 78,
  80–81
  in MBEC for end-of-life elders, 93
  safety reminders for, 187–188

Baby boomers, 6
Barkan, Barry, 163, 164
Bodhi, B., 86
Body scan, 22
  guided meditation, 182–184
  as MBEC group skill, 60–61

as MBEC isolated elder skill, 90
in MBSR professional caregivers
  class, 154
The Breath. *See also* Deep breathing;
  Diaphragmatic breathing
  in CAM dementia interventions,
  77, 80
  in guided meditations, 181–182
  in MBEC for end-of-life elders, 93
  in MBEC informal caregiver
  groups, 125
  in MBEC isolated elder skills, 89
  in mindfulness practices, 20–22
  in yoga, 21–22

CAM. *See* Complementary and
  alternative medicine
CAM dementia interventions. *See also*
  MBEC dementia groups
  aromatherapy as, 78, 80–81
  breathing exercises as, 77, 80
  guided imagery as, 78–79, 80
  hand massage as, 78, 80
  movement as, 79–80
  study of, 80–82
Care recipients, 110, 115, 121
Caregiver groups. *See* MBEC informal
  caregiver groups
Caregivers, 109–111. *See also* Informal
  caregivers; Professional caregivers
  dementia and, 75–76